Behavioral Aspects of Sleep Problems in Childhood and Adolescence

Editor

JUDITH A. OWENS

SLEEP MEDICINE CLINICS

www.sleep.theclinics.com

Consulting Editor
TEOFILO LEE-CHIONG Jr

June 2014 • Volume 9 • Number 2

ELSEVIER

1600 John F. Kennedy Boulevard • Suite 1800 • Philadelphia, Pennsylvania, 19103-2899

http://www.theclinics.com

SLEEP MEDICINE CLINICS Volume 9, Number 2
June 2014, ISSN 1556-407X, ISBN-13: 978-0-323-29932-9

Editor: Patrick Manley
Developmental Editor: Donald Mumford

Sleep Medicine Clinics (ISSN 1556-407X) is published quarterly by Elsevier Inc., 360 Park Avenue South, New York, NY 10010-1710. Months of issue are March, June, September and December. Business and Editorial Offices: 1600 John F. Kennedy Blvd., Ste. 1800, Philadelphia, PA 19103-2899. Customer Service Office: 3251 Riverport Lane, Maryland Heights, MO 63043. Periodicals postage paid at New York, NY and additional mailing offices. Subscription prices are $195.00 per year (US individuals), $95.00 (US residents), $406.00 (US institutions), $230.00 (Canadian individuals), $235.00 (foreign individuals), $135.00 (Canadian and foreign residents) and $452.00 (Canadian and foreign institutions). Foreign air speed delivery is included in all *Clinics* subscription prices. All prices are subject to change without notice. **POSTMASTER:** Send change of address to *Sleep Medicine Clinics*, Elsevier Health Sciences Division, Subscription Customer Service, 3251 Riverport Lane, Maryland Heights, MO 63043. Customer Service: **Tel: 1-800-654-2452 (U.S. and Canada); 314-447-8871 (outside U.S. and Canada). Fax: 314-447-8029. E-mail: journalscustomerservice-usa@elsevier.com (for print support); journalsonlinesupport-usa@elsevier.com (for online support).**

Reprints. For copies of 100 or more of articles in this publication, please contact the Commercial Reprints Department, Elsevier Inc., 360 Park Avenue South, New York, NY 10010-1710. Tel.: 212-633-3874; Fax: 212-633-3820; E-mail: reprints@elsevier.com.

PROGRAM OBJECTIVE

The goal of *Sleep Clinics of North America* is to keep practicing physicians up to date with current clinical practice by providing timely articles reviewing the state of the art in patient care.

TARGET AUDIENCE

All practicing physicians and other healthcare professionals.

LEARNING OBJECTIVES

Upon completion of this activity, participants will be able to:
1. Explain therapies for the improvement of sleep disordered breathing.
2. Review the impact of neurodevelopmental disorders on childhood sleep.
3. Discuss strategies and controversies in treatment of behavioral sleep problems in young children.

ACCREDITATION

The Elsevier Office of Continuing Medical Education (EOCME) is accredited by the Accreditation Council for Continuing Medical Education (ACCME) to provide continuing medical education for physicians.

The EOCME designates this enduringmaterial for a maximum of 15 *AMA PRA Category 1 Credit*(s)™. Physicians should claim only the credit commensurate with the extent of their participation in the activity.

All other health care professionals requesting continuing education credit for this enduring material will be issued a certificate of participation.

DISCLOSURE OF CONFLICTS OF INTEREST

The EOCME assesses conflict of interest with its instructors, faculty, planners, and other individuals who are in a position to control the content of CME activities. All relevant conflicts of interest that are identified are thoroughly vetted by EOCME for fair balance, scientific objectivity, and patient care recommendations. EOCME is committed to providing its learners with CME activities that promote improvements or quality in healthcare and not a specific proprietary business or a commercial interest.

The planning committee, staff, authors and editors listed below have identified no financial relationships or relationships to products or devices they or their spouse/life partner have with commercial interest related to the content of this CME activity:
Candice A. Alfano, PhD; Bjørn Bjorvatn, MD, PhD; Luis F. Buenaver, PhD; Michelle A. Clementi, BS; Penny Corkum, PhD; Jennifer Cowie, BA; Fiona D. Davidson, MASP; Patrick H. Finan, PhD; Kristen Helm; Kerry Holland; Brynne Hunter; Michelle S. King, MD; Brett R. Kuhn, PhD, CBSM; Sandy Lavery; Michel Lecendreux, MD; Daniel S. Lewin, PhD, DABSM, CBSm; Carole L. Marcus, MBBCh; Jill McNair; Jodi A. Mindell, PhD; Melisa Moore, PhD; Mahalakshmi Narayanan; Judith A. Owens, MD, MPH; Michelle A. Patriquin, PhD; Katharine C. Reynolds, BA; Virginia T. Runko, PhD; Marcel G. Smits, MD, PhD; Patrick Sorenson, MA, RPSGT; David Talavera, BA; Kim Tan-MacNeill, BA; Jocelyn H. Thomas, PhD; Shelly K. Weiss, MD, FRCPC; Melissa S. Xanthopoulos, PhD.

The planning committee, staff, authors and editors listed below have identified financial relationships or relationships to products or devices they or their spouse/life partner have with commercial interest related to the content of this CME activity:
Michael L. Gelb, DDS, MS is on speakers bureau for Biolase.
Michael Gradisar, PhD has research grant from Re-Time PTY, Ltd.
Teofilo Lee-Chiong, Jr, MD has stock ownership, a research grant and an employment affiliation with Philips Respironics; is a consultant/advisor for CareCore National and Elsevier; and has royalties/patents with Elsevier, Lippincott, Wiley, Oxford University and CreateSpace.
Joy L. Moeller, RDH, BS is on speakers bureau for AOMT.
Licia Coceani Paskay, MS, CCC-SLP is on speakers bureau for AOMT; and is a consultant/advisor for AOMT and AAMS.
Michael T. Smith, PhD has stock ownership in BMED Interactive.

UNAPPROVED/OFF-LABEL USE DISCLOSURE

The EOCME requires CME faculty to disclose to the participants:
1. When products or procedures being discussed are off-label, unlabelled, experimental, and/or investigational (not US Food and Drug Administration (FDA) approved); and
2. Any limitations on the information presented, such as data that are preliminary or that represent ongoing research, interim analyses, and/or unsupported opinions. Faculty may discuss information about pharmaceutical agents that is outside of FDA-approved labelling. This information is intended solely for CME and is not intended to promote off-label use of these medications. If you have any questions, contact the medical affairs department of the manufacturer for the most recent prescribing information.

TO ENROLL

To enroll in the Sleep Medicines Clinic Continuing Medical Education program, call customer service at 1-800-654-2452 or sign up online at http://www.theclinics.com/home/cme. The CME program is available to subscribers for an additional annual fee of USD $126.

METHOD OF PARTICIPATION

In order to claim credit, participants must complete the following:
1. Complete enrolment as indicated above.
2. Read the activity.
3. Complete the CME Test and Evaluation. Participants must achieve a score of 70% on the test. All CME Tests and Evaluations must be completed online.

CME INQUIRIES/SPECIAL NEEDS

For all CME inquiries or special needs, please contact elsevierCME@elsevier.com.

SLEEP MEDICINE CLINICS

Contributors

CONSULTING EDITOR

TEOFILO LEE-CHIONG Jr, MD
Professor of Medicine, Division of Pulmonary, Critical Care and Sleep Medicine, Department of Medicine, National Jewish Health, University of Colorado, Denver, Colorado; Chief Medical Liaison, Philips Respironics, Pennsylvania

EDITOR

JUDITH A. OWENS, MD, MPH
Director of Sleep Medicine, Division of Pulmonary and Sleep Medicine, Children's National Medical Center, Washington, DC; Professor of Pediatrics, George Washington University School of Medicine and Health Sciences, Washington, DC

AUTHORS

CANDICE A. ALFANO, PhD
Associate Professor, Department of Psychology, University of Houston; Program Director, Sleep and Anxiety Center for Kids (SACK), University of Houston, Houston, Texas

BJØRN BJORVATN, MD, PhD
Professor, Department of Global Public Health and Primary Care, Norwegian Competence Center for Sleep Disorders, Haukeland University Hospital, University of Bergen, Bergen, Norway

LUIS F. BUENAVER, PhD
Assistant Professor, Department of Psychiatry and Behavioral Sciences, Johns Hopkins University School of Medicine, Baltimore, Maryland

MICHELLE A. CLEMENTI, BS
Clinical Psychology Graduate Student, Department of Psychology, University of Houston, Houston, Texas

PENNY CORKUM, PhD
Registered Psychologist; Professor, Clinical Psychology Program, Departments of Psychology and Neuroscience, Psychiatry & Pediatrics, Dalhousie University; Scientific Staff, IWK Health Centre; Director, Attention Deficit/Hyperactivity Disorder Clinic, Colchester East Hants Health Authority, Nova Scotia, Canada

JENNIFER COWIE, BA
Clinical Psychology Graduate Student, Department of Psychology, University of Houston, Houston, Texas

FIONA D. DAVIDSON, MASP
Clinical Psychology PhD Student, Department of Psychology and Neuroscience, Dalhousie University, Halifax, Nova Scotia, Canada

PATRICK H. FINAN, PhD
Assistant Professor, Department of Psychiatry and Behavioral Sciences, Johns Hopkins University School of Medicine, Baltimore, Maryland

MICHAEL L. GELB, DDS, MS
Clinical Professor, Department of
Oral Medicine and Pathology; Clinical
Assistant Professor, Tufts University
School of Dental Medicine, NYU, New York,
New York

MICHAEL GRADISAR, PhD
Associate Professor, School of Psychology,
Flinders University, Adelaide, South Australia,
Australia

MICHELLE S. KING, MD
Sleep Fellow, Sleep Center, The Children's
Hospital of Philadelphia, Perelman School of
Medicine, University of Pennsylvania,
Philadelphia, Pennsylvania

BRETT R. KUHN, PhD, CBSM
Licensed Psychologist and Certified;
Behavioral Sleep Medicine, Associate
Professor, Department of Pediatrics &
Psychology, Munroe-Meyer Institute for
Genetics and Rehabilitation, University of
Nebraska Medical Center, Omaha,
Nebraska

MICHEL LECENDREUX, MD
Pediatric Sleep Center, Hospital Robert
Debré, Paris; National Reference Centre for
Orphan Diseases, Narcolepsy, Idiopathic
Hypersomnia and Kleine-Levin Syndrome
(CNR Narcolepsie-Hypersomnie),
France

DANIEL S. LEWIN, PhD, DABSM, CBSM
Assistant Professor of Pediatrics; Associate
Director, Pediatric Sleep Medicine, Children's
National Medical Center, Washington, DC

CAROLE L. MARCUS, MBBCh
Director of Sleep Center, Sleep Center, The
Children's Hospital of Philadelphia, Perelman
School of Medicine; Professor of Pediatrics,
University of Pennsylvania, Philadelphia,
Pennsylvania

JODI A. MINDELL, PhD
Associate Director, Sleep Center, Division of
Pulmonary Medicine, Children's Hospital of
Philadelphia; Professor, Department of
Psychology, Saint Joseph's University,
Philadelphia, Pennsylvania

JOY L. MOELLER, BS, RDH
Clinical Instructor for the Academy of
Orofacial Myofunctional Therapy (AOMT),
Pacific Palisades, California

MELISA MOORE, PhD
Sleep Center, Division of Pulmonary Medicine,
Children's Hospital of Philadelphia,
Philadelphia, Pennsylvania

JUDITH A. OWENS, MD, MPH
Director of Sleep Medicine, Division of
Pulmonary and Sleep Medicine, Children's
National Medical Center, Washington, DC;
Professor of Pediatrics, George Washington
University School of Medicine and Health
Sciences, Washington, DC

LICIA COCEANI PASKAY, MS, CCC-SLP
Clinical Instructor for the Academy of
Orofacial Myofunctional Therapy (AOMT),
Pacific Palisades, California

MICHELLE A. PATRIQUIN, PhD
Postdoctoral Fellow, Department of
Psychology, Sleep and Anxiety Center for
Kids (SACK), University of Houston, Houston,
Texas

KATHARINE C. REYNOLDS, BA
Clinical Psychology Graduate Student,
Department of Psychology, University of
Houston, Houston, Texas

VIRGINIA T. RUNKO, PhD
Clinical Associate, Department of Psychiatry
and Behavioral Sciences, Johns Hopkins
University School of Medicine, Baltimore,
Maryland

MICHAEL T. SMITH, PhD
Professor, Department of Psychiatry and
Behavioral Sciences, Johns Hopkins
University School of Medicine, Baltimore,
Maryland

MARCEL G. SMITS, MD, PhD
Neurologist and Somnologist, Department of
Neurology, Hospital Gelderse Vallei, Centre for
Sleep-Wake Disorders and Chronobiology,
Ede, The Netherlands

PATRICK SORENSON, MA, RPSGT
Manager, Sleep Laboratory, Department of Sleep Medicine, Children's National Medical Center, Washington, DC

DAVID TALAVERA, BA
Clinical Psychology Graduate Student, Department of Psychology, University of Houston, Houston, Texas

KIM TAN-MACNEILL, BA
Clinical Psychology PhD Student, Department of Psychology and Neuroscience, Dalhousie University, Halifax, Nova Scotia, Canada

JOCELYN H. THOMAS, PhD
Sleep Center, Division of Pulmonary Medicine, Children's Hospital of Philadelphia, Philadelphia, Pennsylvania

SHELLY K. WEISS, MD, FRCPC
Associate Professor, Department of Pediatrics, Hospital for Sick Children, University of Toronto, Toronto, Ontario, Canada

MELISSA S. XANTHOPOULOS, PhD
CPAP Co-ordinator, Sleep Center, The Children's Hospital of Philadelphia, Perelman School of Medicine, University of Pennsylvania, Philadelphia, Pennsylvania

Contents

Sleep problems are a common symptom of childhood anxiety disorders, and can
also exacerbate symptoms of daytime anxiety. Despite evidence for the role of early
sleep disturbance in the development and maintenance of anxiety, research examining the bidirectional relationships underlying these childhood problems is only beginning to emerge. Likewise, intervention components for sleep and anxiety in youth
overlap considerably, yet systematic investigation of combined outcomes is rare.
This article reviews available sleep-focused research in clinically anxious children
and highlights several modifiable targets for early intervention, and presents a newly
developed combined intervention for anxiety and sleep in school-aged children.

Sleep problems represent a troubling aspect for many children with neurodevelopmental disorders (NDD). Prevalence rates of sleep problems range between 50%
and 95% for children with NDD. Given that poor sleep in children with NDD is associated with impairments in daytime functioning, decreased quality of life, increased
NDD symptoms and morbidity, and negative effects on caregivers' health and parenting abilities, these rates are concerning and underscore the need for appropriate
screening, diagnostic evaluation, and management of sleep problems. Behavioral
interventions have empiric support and should be recommended as first-line treatment of sleep problems in this population.

The prevalence rates of insomnias during childhood and adolescence may be
comparable with adult prevalence rates; however, there are no estimates and no
consensus on definitions of insomnia in children 6 years of age and older. There
have been few treatment studies focused on with child and adolescent insomnia.
This article draws on clinical experience and relevant literature in adults and in children less than 6 years of age. Proposed definitions and pathophysiology of child and
adolescent insomnia are described to facilitate treatment planning and as an initial
step toward developing future research.

Empirically based treatments for young children with bedtime refusal and frequent
night-waking have been often and fully described. The goal of this article was
to move beyond the empirically based treatments to discuss additive and

complementary interventions, and provide suggestions for treatment selection, sequencing, and delivery. Clinicians can build on the evidence-based approaches by identifying past treatment failures, creating a sleep-compatible bedroom environment, managing the sleep-wake schedule, optimizing parent-child interactions, adding reinforcement-based strategies, and addressing daytime behaviors or skill deficits that translate to improved child sleep.

This article addresses the treatment of delayed sleep phase disorder (DSPD) in adolescents. As most of the previous literature on this disorder has been tailored primarily to young adults, the focus herein is on adolescents living in the "iEra" and the subjective experience of the adolescent with DSPD. New assessment methods of circadian misalignment, in addition to new medications and devices intended to advance sleep timing, are discussed. Preliminary evidence for the use of psychological therapies to augment classic chronobiological treatments for DSPD is presented.

Narcolepsy is a chronic and disabling neurologic disorder that affects sleep and wakefulness and is characterized by excessive daytime sleepiness, sudden sleep episodes, and attacks of muscle atonia mostly triggered by emotions (cataplexy). Narcolepsy is a lifelong nonprogressive disorder, the onset of which occurs not infrequently during childhood. However, narcolepsy in children is frequently underdiagnosed or misdiagnosed. Young patients affected by the disorder often show dramatic and abrupt impairment in their social skills and academic performance because of excessive daytime sleepiness, fatigue, and lack of energy. Underrecognition and undertreatment of narcolepsy represents a significant unmet medical need in childhood.

Adenotonsillectomy is considered the first-line treatment for obstructive sleep apnea syndrome (OSAS), although not all patients are surgical candidates and some continue to have symptoms after surgery. Positive airway pressure is effective in treating OSAS in these patients by pneumatically splinting the upper airway. Its efficacy is predicated on using the device as prescribed, but adherence is difficult to achieve in both adults and children. Numerous factors are thought to contribute to PAP nonadherence in children. Measures proposed to overcome barriers to adherence include child/parent engagement in PAP treatment, education regarding potential side effects, troubleshooting support, and specific behavioral interventions.

Orofacial myofunctional therapy (OMT) restores nasal breathing and repatterns muscles to correct and optimize the same orofacial functions that are involved in sleep-disordered breathing (SDB). This article explores the link between orofacial muscle dysfunction and SDB and examines the rationale to include OMT in the range of options for pediatric SDB treatments. An overview of the current scientific literature addressing application of OMT in pediatric SDB and a review of both assessment and therapy protocols for SDB and the principles of neuroplasticity and muscle function that make OMT a viable option in treating pediatric SDB are also presented.

For sleep laboratories currently accepting or considering accepting pediatric patients, several key aspects of the structure and processes should be considered that will provide the basic underpinnings necessary for a cohesive team approach. This team approach is critical for the successful operation and function of a pediatric sleep laboratory. There is overlap of adult and pediatric polysomnographic processes but fundamental differences exist as well. These differences can be found in environmental and safety conditions, scheduling concerns, and technological approaches and methodologies. Within this framework are key aspects known to provide an accurate and appropriate diagnosis for children with suspected sleep disorders.

Bedtime problems and night wakings are common concerns for parents and physicians caring for young children. Untreated sleep problems may not resolve without intervention. Behavioral interventions are known to effectively treat bedtime problems and night wakings; however, because there is some degree of controversy surrounding these treatments, clinicians may be reluctant to recommend them and parents may find them unacceptable. This article explores the most common controversies regarding the application of behavioral interventions for sleep problems in children. To help guide clinical decision making, the authors present the available empiric evidence regarding commonly expressed concerns.

Special Article

This article summarizes the literature on cognitive-behavioral therapy for insomnia (CBT-I) in patients with comorbid insomnia and chronic pain. An empiric rationale for the development of CBT-I in chronic pain is provided. The 6 randomized controlled trials in this area are described and contrasted. The data suggest that CBT-I for patients with comorbid insomnia and chronic pain produces clinically meaningful improvements in sleep symptoms. Effects on pain are inconsistent, but tend to favor functional measures over pain severity. Hybrid interventions for insomnia and pain have demonstrated feasibility, but additional trials must be conducted to determine the efficacy relative to CBT-I alone.

Preface

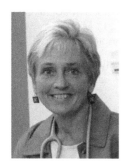

Judith A. Owens, MD, MPH
Editor

It was with great pleasure, mixed with some degree of trepidation, that I accepted the invitation to edit this issue of *Sleep Medicine Clinics*. As a journal editor-in-chief, I well know how challenging it is to convince my overcommitted colleagues to add yet another writing assignment to their already filled-to-overflowing queue. And as a frequent contributor to these types of projects, I also know how difficult it is to say "no," especially to a peer (whom one might in the future ask to return the favor). So I was especially delighted and gratified that all of my invitations to contribute to this issue were graciously accepted. Now that I have seen the results, I am more than grateful and enormously pleased and proud.

The field of pediatric behavioral sleep medicine is one that is truly interdisciplinary, incredibly diverse, and particularly rich in researchers and clinicians with a deep commitment to the health and quality of life of patients and families. This dedication to exemplary patient care, whether it takes the form of evidence-based research, which then informs best practices for the treatment of insomnia in children with anxiety disorders (Alfano and colleagues) or attention deficit hyperactivity disorder (Corkum and colleagues) or reflects the wisdom that comes from years of clinical experience (Kuhn), is the hallmark of what is best about our field. The diversity in perspective of the many disciplines that fall under the pediatric behavioral sleep medicine umbrella and their far-ranging contributions to the treatment of what are traditionally viewed as "medical" sleep disorders is also amply illustrated in this issue. For example, behaviorally based interventions for pediatric sleep disordered breathing include novel approaches such as myofunctional therapy (Moeller and colleagues), strategies to enhance the patient experience in medical diagnostic procedures (Sorenson), and adherence to medical therapies such as positive airway pressure (Marcus and colleagues). Similarly, a refreshing and highly clinically relevant perspective on nonpharmacologic aspects of treatment for one of the few truly "chronic" pediatric sleep disorders, narcolepsy (Lecendreux), bridges the essentially artificial gap between "mental" and "physical" health.

Challenging and adapting the "adult status quo" is another key characteristic of our field, whether that is in reference to the use of cognitive behavior therapy protocols for insomnia in children (Lewin) or the adaptation of behavioral interventions largely developed for and tested in adults for a sleep disorder (delayed sleep wake phase disorder) that actually is most prevalent in the pediatric (ie, adolescent) population (Gradisar and colleagues).

Sleep Med Clin 9 (2014) xiii–xiv
http://dx.doi.org/10.1016/j.jsmc.2014.04.001

And what better example of our field's willingness to embrace divergent views is the candid and thoughtful examination of the controversies that both plague (glass half empty mode) and galvanize (glass full) our field (Mindell and colleagues).

I sincerely hope that you will enjoy reading these contributions as much as I have editing them, and that they will inform your clinical practice and will inspire you to do the much-needed research to advance our field. That having been said, to my colleagues: "I owe you one."

Cheers

Judith A. Owens, MD, MPH
Division of Pulmonary and Sleep Medicine
Children's National Medical Center
111 Michigan Ave NW
Washington DC 20010, USA

George Washington University School of Medicine
and Health Sciences
2300 Eye Street, NW
Washington DC 20037, USA

E-mail address:
owensleep@gmail.com

Addressing Sleep in Children with Anxiety Disorders

Jennifer Cowie, BA[a], Candice A. Alfano, PhD[a,b],*,
Michelle A. Patriquin, PhD[b], Katharine C. Reynolds, BA[a],
David Talavera, BA[a], Michelle A. Clementi, BS[a]

KEYWORDS

- Sleep • Anxiety • Children • Sleep problems • Anxiety disorders • Risk factors • Treatment

KEY POINTS

- The prevalence of sleep problems is more than 90% in some childhood anxiety disorders; however, most data are based on subjective reports, and the specific nature of such problems requires further elucidation.
- A bidirectional relationship between sleep disturbances and anxiety is established, and emerging research is suggestive of numerous pathways and mechanisms through which these problems are interrelated.
- Several theoretically modifiable risk mechanisms, including emotional processing, parenting behaviors, and cognitive factors, hold promise as viable treatment targets.
- Randomized controlled treatment trials for anxious youth have thus far not explored sleep as a potential mediator or outcome of interest. Given the concern that poor sleep may undermine treatment effectiveness by interfering with core treatment components, additional research is clearly needed.

INTRODUCTION

Recognition of the common occurrence of sleep problems in anxious children is not new. Almost a century ago, Denney's[1] description of "The Nervous Child" included acknowledgment of frequent sleep-wake disruption in this population: "*Tiring easily, these children are often so worked up at night by the events of the day that they obtain sleep with difficulty. In the morning they are not refreshed, and are apt to be irritable and peevish during the early hours.*" Decades later, the topic of excessive nighttime fears in children received considerable attention, with multiple studies documenting that symptoms of nighttime disturbances are frequently identified in children with phobias, separation anxiety disorder (SAD), and generalized anxiety disorder (GAD).[2–4] In more recent years, and in conjunction with the development of more reliable measures for evaluating the sleep behaviors of children, sleep-related problems have been reported in up to 90% of children with anxiety disorders.[5–10] Moreover, anxious children who report problems sleeping experience more severe and more impairing anxiety symptoms than do their "good sleeper" counterparts.[6,8]

These important advancements in knowledge notwithstanding, much remains to be learned about the connection between early clinical levels of anxiety and disturbances in the sleep-wake

Conflicts of Interest: None.
[a] Department of Psychology, University of Houston, 126 Heyne Building, Houston, TX 77204, USA;
[b] Department of Psychology, Sleep and Anxiety Center for Kids (SACK), University of Houston, 4505 Cullen Boulevard, Houston, TX 77204, USA
* Corresponding author. Department of Psychology, University of Houston, 126 Heyne Building, Houston, TX 77204.
E-mail address: caalfano@uh.edu

Sleep Med Clin 9 (2014) 137–148
http://dx.doi.org/10.1016/j.jsmc.2014.02.001

cycle. For example, high rates of sleep problems among anxious youth have not yet served to generate systematic research on how sleep might affect treatment, even in the face of experimental findings showing that restricted sleep patterns attenuate reductions in anxiety during treatment.[11–13] Furthermore, although the "sleep problems" of anxious youth have been examined in several investigations, this broad, catch-all term in fact encompasses a diverse range of possible nighttime disturbances ranging from problems initiating sleep, middle-of-the-night awakenings, resistance to or avoidance of getting into bed, and refusal to sleep independently, to shifts in circadian rhythm and parasomnias (eg, sleepwalking, night terrors, enuresis). Understanding of how distinct types of sleep difficulties relate to different forms of anxiety during early development may advance our understanding of mechanisms and dysfunctions of arousal regulation, and contribute to the search for modifiable risk factors.

Sleep disruption is a core feature of anxiety disorders, but the reciprocal nature of these problems must also be emphasized. A host of longitudinal studies highlight childhood sleep problems as an independent prognosticator for the later development of anxiety.[14–16] In one epidemiologic study, for example, close to one-half of school-aged children with persistent sleep problems developed an anxiety diagnosis by the age of 21 years.[15] These data concur with adult-based findings revealing bidirectional temporal relationships between insomnia and anxiety disorders.[17] These types of reciprocal associations are also consistent with results of experimental studies. Specifically, in diverse samples ranging from preschoolers to adults, even modest amounts of experimentally induced sleep restriction reliably produce decreases in positive affect and increases in anxiety/fear.[18–21] Precise mechanisms underlying these relationships are not yet known, but several promising areas of investigation are emerging.

This article provides an overview of the current state of research focused on the sleep of children with anxiety disorders, with an eye toward informing clinical research and prescriptive interventions. The authors begin with an overview of anxiety disorders in youth as described in the Diagnostic and Statistical Manual of Mental Disorders, 5th edition (DSM-5), followed by a review of what is known about the sleep patterns and problems of clinically anxious children. This article focuses closely on 2 specific disorders, in line with available empiric evidence: GAD and SAD. Building on findings from several related lines of research, a few modifiable factors that theoretically could lead to novel ways of addressing these commonly co-occurring problems in children are outlined. Lastly, a newly developed behavioral intervention for anxious children with sleep problems, Targeted Behavioral Therapy or TBT, is described.

OVERVIEW OF CHILDHOOD ANXIETY DISORDERS

Affecting between 8% and 27% of the child population, anxiety disorders are collectively the most prevalent psychiatric conditions in youth.[22] DSM-5[23] includes 7 individual anxiety diagnoses: SAD, GAD, social anxiety disorder, specific phobia, panic disorder, agoraphobia, and selective mutism. Of note, obsessive compulsive disorder (OCD) and posttraumatic stress disorder (PTSD), previously considered anxiety disorders in DSM-IV (text revised), have been reclassified within the newest version of the manual.

A core feature across all anxiety disorders is the presence of excessive fear,[23] which is commonly manifested in the form of heightened physiologic (sympathetic) arousal.[24] Behavioral avoidance and cognitive factors are also central features that cause significant distress. Unlike "normal" childhood fears, clinical levels of worry and anxiety are more severe, more pervasive, and chronic, and are associated with significant impairments in daily life including (but not limited to) increased peer-related problems,[25,26] academic difficulties,[25,27] motor and coordination problems,[28] and family dysfunction.[29] Because anxiety disorders often have a familial component, in terms of both heritability and exposure to parental anxiety, the impact of a diagnosis of child anxiety on the family unit may be particularly heightened. The total direct and indirect cost of medical and mental health care for anxious children is 20 times greater than costs experienced by families with nonanxious children,[30] which may in turn contribute to increased levels of family stress.

Anxiety disorders also rarely occur in isolation,[22] and diagnostic criteria for more than 1 other anxiety or mental health disorder, such as depression, are often met. Moreover, these conditions tend to be chronic, with diagnostic retention rates ranging from 20% to 50% depending on a child's age at the time of the diagnosis and the specific anxiety disorder.[31] For example, childhood social anxiety disorder is frequently associated with continuation of symptoms into adolescence.[32] The presence of childhood anxiety not only increases the risk for anxiety and mood disorders[33,34] in adolescence and adulthood, but is also predictive of other mental health problems such as substance use disorder,[32] conduct disorder, and educational underachievement.[35]

SLEEP PRACTICES IN CHILDREN WITH ANXIETY DISORDERS

For the most part, investigations of sleep issues among clinically anxious children have been concerned with nighttime disturbances rather than with sleep practices such as bedtime routines and sleep-wake schedules. However, the extent to which the sleep problems of these children may be (at least partially) mediated by such factors is potentially important in regard of understanding underlying mechanisms and identifying modifiable risk factors. One study that did address sleep practices compared 1-week prospective sleep diaries of children with various anxiety diagnoses with those of healthy controls, and found that anxious youth had later bedtimes and shorter sleep duration on weekday nights. Anxious youth have also been reported to exhibit less consistency between their weekend and weekday sleep schedules.[10] This finding is likely to be relevant, as there is mounting evidence to suggest that, independent of sleep duration, inconsistent sleep-wake schedules and sleep-related practices are linked not only to sleep problems but also to emotional, behavioral, and attentional difficulties in nonanxious children.[33,34,36] For example, in school-aged children, inconsistent bedtimes and the practice of falling asleep in more than 1 location in the home is associated with increased bedtime resistance.[37] Mindell and colleagues[38] showed that increasing the consistency of young children's bedtimes and pre-bed activities results in significant reductions in sleep-onset latency and number of night awakenings, which could in turn lead to improvements in daytime functioning. At a broader level, family disorganization surrounding daily activities has been shown to account for part of the association between sleep and anxiety problems in children.[39]

Temporal associations between early sleep practices and the development of anxiety have similarly been identified. In one longitudinal study, low rhythmicity (ie, consistency of sleep habits/schedules) during childhood significantly predicted adolescent-onset anxiety (and mood) disorders.[40] In another study, the absence of a set bedtime at age 2 years predicted symptoms of anxiety at age 3 years.[41] Thus, although increasing total sleep duration is often a primary focus of clinicians, maintenance of a stable sleep-wake cycle may be equally critical for anxious children who struggle with other regulatory processes (eg, emotion and attentional regulation), particularly because sleep patterns and practices tend to persist over the longer term.[42]

SLEEP PROBLEMS IN CHILDREN WITH ANXIETY DISORDERS

DSM-5 includes sleep problems as possible diagnostic features of SAD and GAD only, but sleep disruption can occur in conjunction with all forms of anxiety. Rates of sleep problems among clinically anxious youth, including children with various forms of anxiety, are high; mixed anxious samples reveal rates of caregiver and child-reported sleep problems in the range of 82% to 95%.[5–10]

Limited but available findings that use objective sleep measures correspond with studies based on subjective reports. In a study comparing children and adolescents with anxiety disorders with depressed and control youth, based on 2 nights of polysomnography (PSG) in a sleep laboratory, anxious youth exhibited significantly longer sleep-onset latencies and a lower percentage of slow-wave sleep in comparison with both depressed and control groups.[43] The anxiety group also had more nocturnal awakenings in the sleep laboratory than did depressed youth. Using actigraphy, Cousins and colleagues[44] assessed the sleep patterns of youth aged 8 to 16 years with primary anxiety disorders (GAD, SAD, or social anxiety disorder), primary major depressive disorder, and healthy controls. Although not the primary focus of the study, sleep-related findings included significantly longer sleep-onset latencies in anxious youth than in controls. Compared with depressed youth, however, the anxious group showed significantly fewer wake minutes after sleep onset (WASO) as well as increased sleep efficiency. Collectively, findings imply that sleep initiation rather than sleep maintenance is a common source of sleep disturbance for anxious youth.

Although not the focus of this review, it is notable that research focused on children with primary sleep disorders also provides evidence of high rates of comorbid anxiety. In one study 75% of adolescents with sleep terrors and/or sleepwalking also had an anxiety disorder,[45] while another study found that 65% of children and adolescents referred for insomnia had previously received an anxiety diagnosis.[46] Children diagnosed with sleep-disordered breathing and obstructive sleep apnea have greater levels of anxiety and depressive symptoms.[47,48] Among the latter group, affective symptoms are significantly reduced following tonsillectomy and adenoidectomy.[49]

Sleep in Children with Generalized Anxiety Disorder

Consistent with adult-based findings, rates of sleep problems vary with the type of childhood anxiety disorder, and specific anxiety diagnoses are associated with specific types of sleep problems.[7] By far the most widely studied disorder in children with regard to sleep is GAD, which is characterized by excessive and poorly controlled anxiety/worry about a variety of issues. Somatic complaints such as muscle aches and abdominal pain also are commonly present. Sleep-related difficulties occur in up to 95% of children with GAD,[5,7] a higher rate than has been found for other disorders including SAD and social anxiety disorder.[7] In comparison with healthy controls, higher rates of insomnia, nightmares, bedtime resistance, daytime tiredness, and shorter sleep duration have been reported.[5–8]

Objective evidence of sleep disturbance in pediatric GAD is more mixed. A previous study from the authors' group using laboratory-based PSG found prolonged sleep-onset latency, reduced latency to rapid eye movement (REM) sleep, decreased sleep efficiency, and increased total REM sleep among (prepubescent) children with GAD in comparison with controls.[50] However, in a more recent study using unattended ambulatory PSG in the home environment, few differences in sleep architecture between these 2 groups were identified.[51] Laboratory-based sleep differences may be explained in part by the presence of a "first-night effect" (ie, increased habituation over time to PSG assessment in the sleep laboratory environment)[52]; however, at least 1 study suggested that an additional PSG night did not seem to help anxious youth adjust to the laboratory setting.[43] The reasons for the observed discrepancy between objective and subjective sleep findings among children with GAD remain unclear; however, these discrepancies are remarkably similar to those found in children with attention-deficit/hyperactivity disorder (ADHD) based on subjective versus objective measures of sleep.[53,54] Several variables that may contribute to the lack of consistent findings across measures deserve further exploration, including the possible role of parental presence at bedtime/during sleep, reporter bias in subjective reports, and distraction from typical worries/fearful thoughts as a function of undergoing sleep assessment (PSG or actigraphy) at home.

Sleep in Children with Separation Anxiety Disorder

Children with SAD also commonly suffer from sleep disturbances with subjective rates similar to those found among youth with GAD.[6–8] SAD is marked by developmentally inappropriate anxiety and distress on separation from a caregiver. As would be expected based on the nature of the disorder, problems sleeping alone or away from home are very common.[6] In fact, among children with SAD, refusal to sleep independently is among the most frequent reasons for referral to an anxiety specialty clinic.[55] Night terrors and nightmares also are common among children with SAD.[7,8,56]

Few objective sleep data are available to corroborate child and parent reports. However, nighttime and sleep-related disturbances in children who fear parental separation should not automatically be viewed as purely behavioral (ie, subjective) in origin. Findings from experimental research indicate that even brief separations from a caregiver elicit exaggerated physiologic responses in children with SAD (based on a range of cardiac, respiratory, and electrodermal measures) and, on reunion with the caregiver, sympathetic arousal is slower to return to baseline levels in comparison with both controls and children with other anxiety disorders.[57] In animal models, there is evidence for alterations in REM sleep among rat and monkey infants following separation from mothers,[58] highlighting the possible role of architectural sleep changes as a contributor to longer-term difficulties with sleep and regulation of emotion. Inasmuch as physiologic hyperarousal and sleep initiation and maintenance are inherently incompatible processes,[59] it is unsurprising that these children exhibit bedtime resistance, difficulties with falling asleep, and prolonged nighttime awakenings.

THEORETICALLY MODIFIABLE MECHANISMS OF RISK

Despite apparent overlap between sleep disturbances and anxiety in youth, the nature and directionality of these relationships are poorly understood. In one innovative study, Cousins and colleagues[44] aimed to elucidate the temporal sequencing of relationships between nighttime sleep and daytime affect using actigraphy and ecologic momentary assessment data collected over a 2-week period in youth with affective disorders (ie, anxiety disorders and depression) or no psychiatric disorder. The nature of these bidirectional relationships differed across the groups. For youth with an anxiety disorder (only), more positive daytime affect (and increases in a positive to negative affect ratio) was associated with less time spent in bed the following night, and less time spent awake at night was associated with less negative mood the following day. For youth with both anxiety disorders and depression, greater total sleep time was associated with more positive mood the next day. Thus, consistent with a wealth of research, better sleep was associated with better daytime affect for youth with affective disorders. Although daytime anxiety and worry were not specifically examined in this study, the investigators hypothesized that positive affect during the day may translate to less time spent in bed worrying and ruminating (ie, time awake in bed) that night. It is clear, overall, that these problems can persist in a cyclic fashion for extended periods of time. Research aimed at delineating specific mechanistic variables linking sleep and anxiety is therefore needed to inform the content and sequencing of effective preventive and interventional methods. Toward this end, several developing and potentially important areas of investigation are highlighted here.

Emotional Processing

The term emotional processing refers to the coordinated, flexible, multisystem responses (ie, subjective appraisals, physiologic reactions, and regulatory behaviors) attributable to a stimulus that holds personal meaning.[60] Individual differences in emotional processing emerge early, and represent critical aspects of both adaptive and maladaptive development.[61–64] At or around 6 years of age, critical advancements in emotional processing include the ability to accurately identify one's own emotional state as well as the emotions of others, to understand that personal interpretations directly mediate emotional responses, and to hide or modify outward expressions of emotion based on social demands.[65–69] Early deficits in these areas are hypothesized to serve as risk factors for the development of anxiety and mood disorders.[70]

Sleep has a profound impact on emotional processing via its effects on the prefrontal cortex (PFC) and affect-related brain structures such as the amygdala.[71–73] Experimental sleep deprivation/restriction results in overly negative interpretations of and heightened reactivity to emotional stimuli,[73] which are accompanied by changes in activity in these areas of the brain as demonstrated by functional neuroimaging.[74] Such negative effects may be especially detrimental for anxious youth who are already prone to exaggerated physiologic responses[57,75] and biases in emotional appraisal via dysfunction of the same structures.[76–78] In children with GAD, for example, functional connectivity between the PFC and amygdala during emotional processing tasks is negatively associated with severity of anxiety.[76,77] Thus, both levels of arousal and emotional-processing deficits may be exacerbated when sleep is insufficient.

Heightened emotional responses are further compounded by altered patterns of functional brain activity whereby the PFC is less able to inhibit or regulate emotional reactions because of inadequate sleep.[73] Investigations of emotion regulation among clinically anxious children indicate less use of adaptive regulation methods in comparison with nonanxious children.[70,79,80] That is, children with anxiety disorders tend to use maladaptive ways of regulating their emotions, including increased behavioral avoidance, excessive reassurance seeking, and less effective problem-solving.[80] The role of sleep has not been directly investigated in the context of emotion regulation among anxious youth, but emotion regulation was found to fully mediate the relationship between anxiety and sleep disturbance in adults with GAD.[81] For patients with GAD in particular, chronic worry can interfere with the transition to and quality of sleep at night, just as diminished control over worry may be a consequence of inadequate or nonrestful sleep. It is particularly critical to examine these relationships in childhood, a time when sleep and emotion-regulatory systems are codeveloping and the opportunities for prevention/intervention are presumably greatest.

Sleep-Related Parenting Behaviors

A caregiver functions as an external regulator of young children's affect and biological rhythms, and provides scaffolding for the development of self-regulation capacities.[82] In broad terms, parental overcontrol, defined as excessive regulation of child behavior and/or encouragement of dependency on parents (ie, lack of autonomy) is proposed to undermine self-efficacy and increase the risk for anxiety.[83] Indeed, this parenting style is more common among anxious children than in children without anxiety disorders.[10] These same parenting behaviors are also positively associated with sleep disruption during early development,[42] presumably by interfering with the development of regulatory skills needed to self-soothe at sleep onset.[84,85] For example, Sheridan and colleagues[86] found that parental overinvolvement in infants' sleep (in the form of active soothing and presence at sleep onset) was associated with sleep problems at age 5 years. Maternal promotion of autonomy at 12 and 15 months of age has been found to correlate significantly with a higher percentage of nighttime sleep in 3- to 4-year-olds.[87]

In a retrospective study among 7- to 11-year-old children, the authors compared early parenting behaviors related to sleep in children with a primary GAD diagnosis and healthy controls.[88] During the first 6 months of life, children with GAD were significantly more likely to be breastfed directly before sleep and to be rocked to sleep at night. In the GAD group, but not among controls, these early sleep practices were significantly associated with current parent-reported sleep problems. Moreover, a history of cosleeping in infancy was significantly positively associated with sleep problems as reported by children with GAD, but not controls. Similar behaviors including overinvolvement in bedtime routines and sharing a room or bed have been found among mothers with panic disorder and separation anxiety,[89,90] which were in turn associated with elevated rates of children's sleep problems. These findings concur with other research[86] to suggest that early sleep-related parenting practices may have a long-term impact on child sleep patterns, and increase (or decrease) the risk for sleep problems. Moreover, differential associations found between parenting behaviors in infancy and sleep in childhood in anxious versus nonanxious children (J. Balderas, D. Talavera, C. Grochet, et al, unpublished data, 2014 [article under review]) highlight the importance of considering temperament-parenting interactions with regard to early sleep practices. From a clinical standpoint, targeting early parenting practices with regard to sleep in families where a parent and/or child exhibits elevated levels of anxiety may be a crucial aspect of early intervention.

Cognitive Factors

Cognitive arousal or excessive cognitive activity/worry at bedtime is a frequent complaint of both anxious adults[91] and individuals with insomnia.[92] Adults with both insomnia and GAD report greater levels of presleep cognitive activity than do insomniacs and good sleepers.[93] Because the ability to self-regulate is still developing in children, excessive mentation at bedtime may be especially difficult to control, and thus could interfere with sleep initiation. This conclusion has been supported by the results of several studies. For example, Gregory and colleagues[94] found that increased cognitive arousal during the presleep period was predictive of parent and child-reported sleep problems in a community sample of children 8 to 10 years old. Among anxious youth,[7] high levels of presleep cognitive arousal have been associated with decreased total sleep duration and increased rates of sleep problems. Common themes of child nighttime fears that could contribute to cognitive arousal include personal safety (eg, intruders), environmental threats (eg, strange noises), and imaginary creatures.[95,96] Investigations exploring the actual content of presleep mentation in children, including those with anxiety disorders, are nonetheless needed.

Building on adult models of insomnia, an individual's cognitive responses to sleep difficulties can serve to maintain or exacerbate sleep problems, and insomnia is more likely to persist if nighttime difficulties are perceived as a sign of threat or a loss of control.[95] This process has been termed "catastrophizing" about the consequences of sleeplessness, and is associated with increased levels of anxiety in adults and adolescents who are poor sleepers.[21,96] Children as young as 8 years also appear to catastrophize about poor sleep and the potential impact of sleep problems on physiologic, emotional, and other aspects of functioning.[97] Catastrophizing about the consequences of negative events, in general, as well as other interpretation biases are commonly found in children with anxiety disorders, and are hypothesized to contribute to the development of these disorders.[98,99] In nonclinical samples, sleep problems correlate significantly with interpretation biases (including catastrophizing), although this association seems to be better accounted for by co-occurring anxiety and depression symptoms.[97,100] Targeting catastrophizing and other dysfunctional cognitive beliefs about sleep may serve to produce enhanced sleep outcomes for youth with clinical levels of anxiety.

ADDRESSING SLEEP PROBLEMS IN CLINICALLY ANXIOUS YOUTH

Despite extensive overlap in risk, remarkably little research has explored sleep as a potential mediator or outcome of interest in randomized controlled trials among clinically anxious youth. Poor sleep may nonetheless undermine treatment effectiveness by interfering with central cognitive and behavioral treatment components requiring self-control, sustained attention, and rehearsal in nonthreatening environments.[101,102] Indeed, behaviors associated with sleep loss in children such as hyperactivity, inattentiveness, and poor impulse control overlap with the cardinal symptoms of ADHD in children,[59] and thus might be expected to impede central goals of treatment. For example, in vivo exposure, a core component of cognitive-behavioral therapy (CBT), requires a child to face a feared stimulus for a sustained period of time while experiencing (uncomfortable) heightened feelings of arousal. Habituation to the feared stimulus, which is the goal of exposure, is unlikely to occur if the child is distracted or physically avoids the task.[103] Thus, owing to decrements in the regulation of attentional, motivational, behavioral, and/or emotional responses,[104,105] exposure tasks may be less likely to result in habituation if sleep problems and/or insufficient sleep are not addressed. Moreover, even when in-session habituation does occur, generalization to similar stimuli outside the clinical setting may be hampered by sleep loss.[11,12,71]

Overlapping Interventions

Behavioral treatments for child anxiety disorders and insomnia share several intersecting components, including avoidance reduction (eg, staying home from school, sleeping with parents), relaxation strategies (eg, for managing daytime and nighttime arousal), and parents' management techniques (eg, encouraging approach behaviors, limiting involvement in bedtime routines).[106,107] Accordingly, treatment gains in one domain may generalize to the other via reductions in arousal, increases in self-regulatory skill, or greater use of approach behaviors.

A few studies have shown brief cognitive-behavioral (eg, 6-session) interventions for insomnia to produce improvements not only in sleep but also in anxiety symptoms among school-aged children.[108,109] On the other hand, only 1 waitlist-controlled CBT treatment trial for childhood anxiety has examined the impact on sleep-based outcomes. CBT resulted in a reduction in postintervention complaints of "sleep disturbances" compared with baseline.[110] However, sleep was not a primary outcome measure in this study and the specific nature of children's sleep disturbances was not explored, so the extent to which CBT produced significant changes in specific sleep parameters is unclear. Overall, this is a preliminary body of research that prompts many more questions as to whether sleep-based improvements are observable following CBT for childhood anxiety or, alternatively, whether the inclusion of sleep-focused intervention components might produce more optimal immediate and long-term outcomes in the treatment of anxiety disorders.

Targeted Behavioral Therapy for Children with GAD

To begin to address these questions, the authors recently developed a manualized treatment targeting both anxiety and sleep problems in children, called Targeted Behavioral Therapy (TBT).[111] TBT was developed for school-aged children with a diagnosis of GAD because of the high prevalence of sleep disturbances in this specific population as well as the reciprocal nature of sleep and anxiety symptoms. However, it is anticipated that this protocol may well be applicable to a broader range of anxious children. Several aspects of TBT are

noteworthy. First, in light of the potential for persistent sleep problems to interfere with core intervention components for anxiety, the 14-session intervention targets sleep knowledge and behaviors at the outset of treatment. Second, although most TBT sessions are delivered in an individual format (ie, the child only), sleep-focused sessions include both parents and children together, highlighting the importance of parents in establishing healthy sleep habits and helping children to develop nighttime self-regulatory strategies. Lastly, TBT enables the clinician to develop a prescriptive approach to treating each child's individual sleep problems. Following sleep-based education, the therapist helps children and parents identify "sleep enemies" present at home, such as inconsistent bed/wake times, engaging in arousing activities before bed, or not sleeping alone in one's own bed; information which is then used to inform an individualized treatment plan. The therapist can then match the child's unique sleep problems to 1 or more intervention strategies outlined in the manual. As an example, for a child who consistently avoids going to bed and requires parental presence at sleep onset because of excessive nighttime fears, a combination of healthy sleep practices, graduated extinction procedures, and self-directed relaxation strategies might be chosen to help the child to learn to go to bed and fall asleep independently.

The authors recently published a case series of 4 children with primary GAD[111] to provide a preliminary examination of the efficacy of TBT. In addition to significant reductions in anxiety and improvements in global functioning, 3 of the 4 children reported clinically meaningful improvements in sleep problems after treatment and at a 3-month follow-up assessment. However, some differences between child and parent sleep reports were observed, in that parents were less likely to endorse improvements following treatment. The reasons for this discrepancy are not entirely clear, but it is possible that some child-reported improvements in sleep occurred without parental awareness (eg, nighttime fears/worries, sleep-onset latency), underscoring the importance of questioning both child and parent about sleep problems. Alternatively, including only 2 sessions focused on sleep may be insufficient for altering sleep patterns and behaviors over the long term. The authors are currently conducting a randomized controlled trial comparing an extended version of TBT (including 2 additional sleep-focused sessions) with an active control treatment, which will allow for a more in-depth evaluation of outcomes using both subjective and objective (actigraphy) sleep assessments.

SUMMARY

Childhood anxiety disorders are highly prevalent and are often associated with significant sleep disturbance. Although data are still somewhat limited and results may vary across different diagnoses, methods, and informants, empirical evidence has begun to emerge to corroborate high rates of subjective sleep complaints in anxious youth, primarily those with GAD. The sleep problems, patterns, and practices of clinically anxious youth represent an important window onto the relationship between sleep and emotional regulation, and may assist in answering questions regarding the relative contributions of sleep-wake schedules versus disruptions to daytime emotional impairments. Research focused on further specifying the types of sleep disturbances experienced by youth with various forms of anxiety is also needed to inform theoretical models and the development of effective interventions.

Multiple mechanisms may well influence acute and long-term relationships between sleep and anxiety, and several factors in particular represent viable targets for clinical research. Overlapping deficits in the processing of emotional information, parenting behaviors that hinder the development of self-regulatory skills, catastrophizing about sleep, and other cognitive biases are common to both sleep-deprived and anxious youth, all or any of which may serve as a functional pathway for the development of these problems. Investigation of such factors may not only inform the content of effective intervention approaches, but may help to instruct the ideal timing and sequencing of such methods, especially as co-occurring sleep disturbance may reduce the effectiveness of anxiety-based treatment modalities. TBT is an example of a novel prescriptive intervention targeting both sleep and anxiety in children with GAD that has demonstrated initial efficacy in both domains, thereby setting the stage for the development of further research.

REFERENCES

1. Denney W. The nervous child. Can Med Assoc J 1928;18(5):555.
2. Connell H, Persley G, Sturgess J. Sleep phobia in middle childhood—a review of six cases. J Am Acad Child Adolesc Psychiatry 1987;26(3):449–52.
3. Graziano AM, DeGiovanni IS, Garcia KA. Behavioral treatment of children's fears: a review. Psychol Bull 1979;86(4):804.
4. King NJ, Hamilton DI, Ollendick TH. Children's phobias: a behavioural perspective. Chichester (United Kingdom): Wiley; 1988.
5. Alfano CA, Beidel DC, Turner SM, et al. Preliminary evidence for sleep complaints among children referred for anxiety. Sleep Med 2006;7(6):467–73.
6. Alfano CA, Ginsburg GS, Kingery JN. Sleep-related problems among children and adolescents with anxiety disorders. J Am Acad Child Adolesc Psychiatry 2007;46(2):224–32.
7. Alfano CA, Pina AA, Zerr AA, et al. Pre-sleep arousal and sleep problems of anxiety-disordered youth. Child Psychiatry Hum Dev 2010;41(2):156–67.
8. Chase RM, Pincus DB. Sleep-related problems in children and adolescents with anxiety disorders. Behav Sleep Med 2011;9(4):224–36.
9. Hansen BH, Skirbekk B, Oerbeck B, et al. Comparison of sleep problems in children with anxiety and attention deficit/hyperactivity disorders. Eur Child Adolesc Psychiatry 2011;20(6):321–30.
10. Hudson JL, Gradisar M, Gamble A, et al. The sleep patterns and problems of clinically anxious children. Behav Res Ther 2009;47(4):339–44.
11. Kleim B, Wilhelm F, Temp L, et al. Sleep enhances exposure therapy. Psychol Med 2013;10:1–9.
12. Pace-Schott EF, Milad MR, Orr SP, et al. Sleep promotes generalization of extinction of conditioned fear. Sleep 2009;32(1):19.
13. Pace-Schott EF, Spencer R, Vijayakumar S, et al. Extinction of conditioned fear is better learned and recalled in the morning than in the evening. J Psychiatr Res 2013;47(11):1776–84.
14. Gregory AM, Eley TC, O'Connor TG, et al. Etiologies of associations between childhood sleep and behavioral problems in a large twin sample. J Am Acad Child Adolesc Psychiatry 2004;43(6):744–51.
15. Gregory AM, Caspi A, Eley TC, et al. Prospective longitudinal associations between persistent sleep problems in childhood and anxiety and depression disorders in adulthood. J Abnorm Child Psychol 2005;33(2):157–63.
16. Johnson EO, Chilcoat HD, Breslau N. Trouble sleeping and anxiety/depression in childhood. Psychiatry Res 2000;94(2):93–102.
17. Ohayon MM, Roth T. Place of chronic insomnia in the course of depressive and anxiety disorders. J Psychiatr Res 2003;37(1):9–15.
18. Berger RH, Miller AL, Seifer R, et al. Acute sleep restriction effects on emotion responses in 30- to 36-month-old children. J Sleep Res 2012;21(3):235–46.
19. Dagys N, McGlinchey EL, Talbot LS, et al. Double trouble? The effects of sleep deprivation and chronotype on adolescent affect. J Child Psychol Psychiatry 2012;53(6):660–7.
20. Dinges DF, Pack F, Williams K, et al. Cumulative sleepiness, mood disturbance and psychomotor

vigilance performance decrements during a week of sleep restricted to 4-5 hours per night. Sleep 1997;20(4):267–77.

21. Talbot LS, McGlinchey EL, Kaplan KA, et al. Sleep deprivation in adolescents and adults: changes in affect. Emotion 2010;10(6):831.

22. Costello EJ, Egger HL, Angold A. Developmental epidemiology of anxiety disorders. In: Ollendick TH, March JS, editors. Phobic and anxiety disorders in children and adolescents: A clinician's guide to effective psychosocial and pharmacological interventions. New York (NY): Oxford University Press; 2004.

23. Association AP. Diagnostic and statistical manual of mental disorders. 5th edition. Washington, DC: Association AP; 2013.

24. Friedman BH. An autonomic flexibility-neurovisceral integration model of anxiety and cardiac vagal tone. Biol Psychol 2007;74(2): 185–99.

25. Strauss CC, Frame CL, Forehand R. Psychosocial impairment associated with anxiety in children. J Clin Child Psychol 1987;16(3):235–9.

26. Strauss CC, Forehand R, Smith K, et al. The association between social withdrawal and internalizing problems of children. J Abnorm Child Psychol 1986;14(4):525–35.

27. Kashani JH, Orvaschel H. A community study of anxiety in children and adolescents. Am J Psychiatry 1990;147(3):313–8.

28. Schoemaker MM, Kalverboer AF. Social and affective problems of children who are clumsy: how early do they begin? Adapt Phys Activ Q 1994; 11:140.

29. Ezpeleta L, Keeler G, Erkanli A, et al. Epidemiology of psychiatric disability in childhood and adolescence. J Child Psychol Psychiatry 2001;42(7): 901–14.

30. Bodden DH, Dirksen CD, Bögels SM. Societal burden of clinically anxious youth referred for treatment: a cost-of-illness study. J Abnorm Child Psychol 2008;36(4):487–97.

31. Beidel DC, Alfano CA. Child anxiety disorders: a guide to research and treatment. New York (NY): Taylor & Francis; 2013.

32. Bittner A, Egger HL, Erkanli A, et al. What do childhood anxiety disorders predict? J Child Psychol Psychiatry 2007;48(12):1174–83.

33. Biggs SN, Lushington K, van den Heuvel CJ, et al. Inconsistent sleep schedules and daytime behavioral difficulties in school-aged children. Sleep Med 2011;12(8):780–6.

34. Sadeh A, Raviv A, Gruber R. Sleep patterns and sleep disruptions in school-age children. Dev Psychol 2000;36(3):291–301.

35. Woodward LJ, Fergusson DM. Life course outcomes of young people with anxiety disorders in adolescence. J Am Acad Child Adolesc Psychiatry 2001;40(9):1086–93.

36. Wolfson AR, Carskadon MA. Sleep schedules and daytime functioning in adolescents. Child Dev 1998;69(4):875–87.

37. Blader JC, Koplewicz HS, Abikoff H, et al. Sleep problems of elementary school children. A community survey. Arch Pediatr Adolesc Med 1997; 151(5):473–80.

38. Mindell JA, Telofski LS, Wiegand B, et al. A nightly bedtime routine: impact on sleep in young children and maternal mood. Sleep 2009; 32(5):599–606.

39. Gregory AM, Eley TC, O'Conner TG, et al. Family influences on the association between sleep problems and anxiety in a large sample of preschool aged twins. Pers Individ Dif 2005;(29): 1337–48.

40. Ong SH, Wickramaratne P, Tang M, et al. Early childhood sleep and eating problems as predictors of adolescent and adult mood and anxiety disorders. J Affect Disord 2006;96(1):1–8.

41. Jansen PW, Saridjan NS, Hofman A, et al. Does disturbed sleeping precede symptoms of anxiety or depression in toddlers? The generation R study. Psychosom Med 2011;73(3):242–9.

42. Klackenberg G. Sleep behaviour studied longitudinally. Data from 4-16 years on duration, night-awakening and bed-sharing. Acta Paediatr Scand 1982;71(3):501–6.

43. Forbes EE, Bertocci MA, Gregory AM, et al. Objective sleep in pediatric anxiety disorders and major depressive disorder. J Am Acad Child Adolesc Psychiatry 2008;47(2):148–55.

44. Cousins JC, Whalen DJ, Dahl RE, et al. The bidirectional association between daytime affect and nighttime sleep in youth with anxiety and depression. J Pediatr Psychol 2011;36(9):969–79.

45. Gau SF, Soong WT. Psychiatric comorbidity of adolescents with sleep terrors or sleepwalking: a case-control study. Aust N Z J Psychiatry 1999;33(5): 734–9.

46. Ivanenko A, Barnes ME, Crabtree VM, et al. Psychiatric symptoms in children with insomnia referred to a pediatric sleep medicine center. Sleep Med 2004;5(3):253–9.

47. Rosen CL, Storfer-Isser A, Taylor HG, et al. Increased behavioral morbidity in school-aged children with sleep-disordered breathing. Pediatrics 2004;114(6):1640–8.

48. O'Brien LM, Mervis CB, Holbrook CR, et al. Neurobehavioral implications of habitual snoring in children. Pediatrics 2004;114(1):44–9.

49. Goldstein NA, Fatima M, Campbell TF, et al. Child behavior and quality of life before and after tonsillectomy and adenoidectomy. Arch Otolaryngol Head Neck Surg 2002;128(7):770–5.

50. Alfano CA, Reynolds K, Scott N, et al. Polysomnographic sleep patterns of non-depressed, non-medicated children with generalized anxiety disorder. J Affect Disord 2013;147(1–3): 379–84.

51. Patriquin MA, Mellman TA, Glaze DG, et al. Polysomnographic sleep characteristics of generally-anxious and healthy children assessed in the home environment. J Affect Disord, in press.

52. Agnew HW, Webb WB, Williams RL. The first night effect: an EEG study of sleep. Psychophysiology 1966;2(3):263–6.

53. Moreau V, Rouleau N, Morin CM. Sleep of children with attention deficit hyperactivity disorder: actigraphic and parental reports. Behav Sleep Med 2014;12(1):69–83.

54. Owens J, Gruber R, Brown T, et al. Future research directions in sleep and ADHD report of a Consensus Working Group. J Atten Disord 2013; 17(7):550–64.

55. Eisen AR, Schaefer CE. Separation anxiety in children and adolescents: an individualized approach to assessment and treatment. New York (NY): Guilford Press; 2005.

56. Verduin TL, Kendall PC. Differential occurrence of comorbidity within childhood anxiety disorders. J Clin Child Adolesc Psychol 2003;32(2): 290–5.

57. Kossowsky J, Wilhelm FH, Roth WT, et al. Separation anxiety disorder in children: disorder-specific responses to experimental separation from the mother. J Child Psychol Psychiatry 2012;53(2): 178–87.

58. McKenna J, Mosko S, Richard C, et al. Experimental studies of infant-parent co-sleeping: mutual physiological and behavioral influences and their relevance to SIDS (sudden infant death syndrome). Early Hum Dev 1994;38(3):187–201.

59. Dahl RE. The regulation of sleep and arousal: development and psychopathology. Dev Psychopathol 1996;8:3–28.

60. Gross JJ, Thompson RA. Emotion regulation: Conceptual foundations. In: Gross JJ, editor. Handbook of emotion regulation. New York (NY): Guilford Press; 2007.

61. Eisenberg N, Cumberland A, Spinrad TL, et al. The relations of regulation and emotionality to children's externalizing and internalizing problem behavior. Child Dev 2001;72(4):1112–34.

62. Rubin KH, Coplan RJ, Fox NA, et al. Emotionality, emotion regulation, and preschoolers' social adaptation. Dev Psychopathol 1995;7:49.

63. Sheeber L, Allen N, Davis B, et al. Regulation of negative affect during mother-child problem-solvinginteractions: adolescent depressive status and family processes. J Abnorm Child Psychol 2000;28(5):467–79.

64. Silk JS, Steinberg L, Morris AS. Adolescents' emotion regulation in daily life: links to depressive symptoms and problem behavior. Child Dev 2003; 74(6):1869–80.

65. Banerjee M. Hidden emotions: preschoolers' knowledge of appearance-reality and emotion display rules. Soc Cognit 1997;15(2):107–32.

66. Bradmetz J, Schneider R. Is Little Red Riding Hood afraid of her grandmother? Cognitive vs. emotional response to a false belief. Br J Dev Psychol 1999; 17(4):501–14.

67. Harris PL, Johnson CN, Hutton D, et al. Young children's theory of mind and emotion. Cognit Emot 1989;3(4):379–400.

68. Herba CM, Landau S, Russell T, et al. The development of emotion-processing in children: effects of age, emotion, and intensity. J Child Psychol Psychiatry 2006;47(11):1098–106.

69. Posner MI, Rothbart MK. Developing mechanisms of self-regulation. Dev Psychopathol 2000;12(3): 427–41.

70. Suveg C, Zeman J. Emotion regulation in children with anxiety disorders. J Clin Child Adolesc Psychol 2004;33(4):750–9.

71. Pace-Schott EF, Nave G, Morgan A, et al. Sleep-dependent modulation of affectively guided decision-making. J Sleep Res 2012;21(1):30–9.

72. Thomas M, Sing H, Belenky G, et al. Neural basis of alertness and cognitive performance impairments during sleepiness. I. Effects of 24 h of sleep deprivation on waking human regional brain activity. J Sleep Res 2000;9(4):335–52.

73. Yoo SS, Gujar N, Hu P, et al. The human emotional brain without sleep—a prefrontal amygdala disconnect. Curr Biol 2007;17(20):R877–8.

74. van der Helm E, Gujar N, Walker MP. Sleep deprivation impairs the accurate recognition of human emotions. Sleep 2010;33(3):335–42.

75. Weems CF, Zakem AH, Costa NM, et al. Physiological response and childhood anxiety: association with symptoms of anxiety disorders and cognitive bias. J Clin Child Adolesc Psychol 2005;34(4): 712–23.

76. McClure EB, Monk CS, Nelson EE, et al. Abnormal attention modulation of fear circuit function in pediatric generalized anxiety disorder. Arch Gen Psychiatry 2007;64(1):97.

77. Monk C, Nelson E, McClure E, et al. Ventrolateral prefrontal cortex activation and attentional bias in response to angry faces in adolescents with generalized anxiety disorder. Am J Psychiatry 2006; 163(6):1091–7.

78. Monk CS, Telzer EH, Mogg K, et al. Amygdala and ventrolateral prefrontal cortex activation to masked angry faces in children and adolescents with generalized anxiety disorder. Arch Gen Psychiatry 2008;65(5):568.

79. Carthy T, Horesh N, Apter A, et al. Emotional reactivity and cognitive regulation in anxious children. Behav Res Ther 2010;48(5):384–93.

80. Carthy T, Horesh N, Apter A, et al. Patterns of emotional reactivity and regulation in children with anxiety disorders. J Psychopathol Behav Assess 2010;32(1):23–36.

81. Tsypes A, Aldao A, Mennin DS. Emotion dysregulation and sleep difficulties in generalized anxiety disorder. J Anxiety Disord 2013;27(2):197–203.

82. Anders TF. Infant sleep, nighttime relationships, and attachment. Psychiatry 1994;57(1):11–21.

83. Wood JJ. Parental intrusiveness and children's separation anxiety in a clinical sample. Child Psychiatry Hum Dev 2006;37(1):73–87.

84. Sadeh A, Tikotzky L, Scher A. Parenting and infant sleep. Sleep Med Rev 2010;14(2):89–96.

85. Alfano CA, Smith VC, Reynolds KC, et al. The Parent-Child Sleep Interactions Scale (PSIS) for preschoolers: factor structure and initial psychometric properties. J Clin Sleep Med 2013;9(11):1153–60.

86. Sheridan A, Murray L, Cooper PJ, et al. A longitudinal study of child sleep in high and low risk families: relationship to early maternal settling strategies and child psychological functioning. Sleep Med 2013;14(3):266–73.

87. Bordeleau S, Bernier A, Carrier J. Longitudinal associations between the quality of parent-child interactions and children's sleep at preschool age. J Fam Psychol 2012;26(2):254–62.

88. Balderas J, Talavera D, Grochet C, et al. Sleep-related parenting behaviors during infancy are associated with sleep problems in generalized anxiety disorder of childhood. [Manuscript in preparation].

89. Scher A. Maternal separation anxiety as a regulator of infants' sleep. J Child Psychol Psychiatry 2008;49(6):618–25.

90. Warren SL, Gunnar MR, Kagan J, et al. Maternal panic disorder: infant temperament, neurophysiology, and parenting behaviors. J Am Acad Child Adolesc Psychiatry 2003;42(7):814–25.

91. Monti JM, Monti D. Sleep disturbance in generalized anxiety disorder and its treatment. Sleep Med Rev 2000;4(3):263–76.

92. Riemann D, Spiegelhalder K, Feige B, et al. The hyperarousal model of insomnia: a review of the concept and its evidence. Sleep Med Rev 2010;14(1):19–31.

93. Belanger L, Morin CM, Gendron L, et al. Presleep cognitive activity and thought control strategies in insomnia. J Cognit Psychother 2005;19(1):19–28.

94. Gregory AM, Willis TA, Wiggs L, et al. Presleep arousal and sleep disturbances in children. Sleep 2008;31(12):1745–7.

95. Morin CM, Stone J, Trinkle D, et al. Dysfunctional beliefs and attitudes about sleep among older adults with and without insomnia complaints. Psychol Aging 1993;8(3):463.

96. Harvey AG, Greenall E. Catastrophic worry in primary insomnia. J Behav Ther Exp Psychiatry 2003;34(1):11–23.

97. Gregory AM, Noone DM, Eley TC, et al. Catastrophizing and symptoms of sleep disturbances in children. J Sleep Res 2010;19(1 Pt 2):175–82.

98. Weems CF, Berman SL, Silverman WK, et al. Cognitive errors in youth with anxiety disorders: the linkages between negative cognitive errors and anxious symptoms. Cognit Ther Res 2001;25(5):559–75.

99. Weems CF, Costa NM, Watts SE, et al. Cognitive errors, anxiety sensitivity, and anxiety control beliefs their unique and specific associations with childhood anxiety symptoms. Behav Modif 2007;31(2):174–201.

100. Alfano CA, Gamble AL. The role of sleep in childhood psychiatric disorders. Child Youth Care Forum 2009;38(6):327–40.

101. Delaney KR, Hawkins-Walsh E. Cognitive and behavioral approaches in child and adolescent mental health treatment. In: Yearwood EL, Pearson GS, Newland JA, editors. Child and Adolescent Behavioral Health. West Sussex (UK): John Wiley & Sons; 2012.

102. Hannesdottir DK, Ollendick TH. The role of emotion regulation in the treatment of child anxiety disorders. Clin Child Fam Psychol Rev 2007;10(3):275–93.

103. Abramowitz JS, Deacon BJ, Whiteside SP. Exposure therapy for anxiety: principles and practice. New York (NY): Guilford Press; 2012.

104. Dahl RE, Lewin DS. Pathways to adolescent health sleep regulation and behavior. J Adolesc Health 2002;31(6):175–84.

105. Sadeh A, Gruber R, Raviv A. The effects of sleep restriction and extension on school-age children: what a difference an hour makes. Child Dev 2003;74(2):444–55.

106. Silverman WK, Pina AA, Viswesvaran C. Evidence-based psychosocial treatments for phobic and anxiety disorders in children and adolescents. J Clin Child Adolesc Psychol 2008;37(1):105–30.

107. Clementi M, Balderas J, Cowie J, et al, editors. Behavioral treatment of childhood insomnia. In: Alfano CA, Beidel DC, editors. Comprehensive evidence-based interventions for school-aged children and adolescents. Hoboken (NJ): Wiley; in press.

108. Paine S, Gradisar M. A randomised controlled trial of cognitive-behaviour therapy for behavioural insomnia of childhood in school-aged children. Behav Res Ther 2011;49(6–7):379–88.

109. Schlarb AA, Velten-Schurian K, Poets CF, et al. First effects of a multicomponent treatment for sleep disorders in children. Nat Sci Sleep 2011; 3:1.

110. Kendall PC, Pimentel SS. On the physiological symptom constellation in youth with generalized anxiety disorder (GAD). J Anxiety Disord 2003; 17(2):211–21.

111. Clementi MA, Alfano CA. Targeted behavioral therapy for childhood generalized anxiety disorder: a time-series analysis of changes in anxiety and sleep. J Anxiety Disord 2014;28(2):215–22.

Sleep in Children with Neurodevelopmental Disorders
A Focus on Insomnia in Children with ADHD and ASD

Penny Corkum, PhD[a,b,c,d],*, Fiona D. Davidson, MASP[e],
Kim Tan-MacNeill, BA[e], Shelly K. Weiss, MD, FRCPC[f]

KEYWORDS

- Pediatric • Sleep • Insomnia • Assessment • Treatment

KEY POINTS

- Sleep disturbances affect between 50% and 95% of children with neurodevelopmental disorders (NDD), with behavioral insomnia the most common problem.
- Behavioral insomnia in children with NDD is associated with impairments in daytime functioning, decreased quality of life for the children, and negative effects on caregivers' health and parenting and adds to the morbidity of NDD; thus, appropriate screening, evaluation, and management of sleep problems can have a significant impact on quality of life in these children and families.
- Behavioral interventions have been shown an effective insomnia treatment strategy in typically developing (TD) children, and there is emerging empiric evidence that they are also effective for children with NDD.
- Children with NDD may require modifications to the ways in which behavioral insomnia is typically assessed and managed.
- Currently, there are no recommended pharmacologic treatments for managing behavioral insomnia in children with NDD, although there is mounting research for the effectiveness of melatonin for treating sleep-onset problems in children with attention-deficit/hyperactivity disorder (ADHD).

INTRODUCTION

Sleep is important for the healthy development for all children, yet sleep problems are common, affecting approximately 20% to 30% of TD children.[1] The most common sleep problems are often primarily behavioral in nature and include bedtime resistance, difficulty falling asleep, night wakings, and early morning awakenings, all of which can shorten sleep duration.[2] Collectively, these behavioral problems that have an impact on sleep may be categorized as *behavioral insomnia*, which is the focus of this article.

Disclosure Statement: None of the authors has any conflicts of interest in relation to the submitted article.
[a] Clinical Psychology Program, Department of Psychology and Neuroscience, Dalhousie University, Halifax, Nova Scotia, Canada; [b] Department of Psychiatry, Dalhousie University, Halifax, Nova Scotia, Canada; [c] Department of Pediatrics, Dalhousie University, Halifax, Nova Scotia, Canada; [d] Attention Deficit/Hyperactivity Disorder Clinic, Colchester East Hants Health Authority, Truro, Nova Scotia, Canada; [e] Department of Psychology and Neuroscience, Dalhousie University, Halifax, Nova Scotia, Canada; [f] Department of Pediatrics, Hospital for Sick Children, University of Toronto, Toronto, Ontario, Canada
* Corresponding author. Department of Psychology & Neuroscience, Dalhousie University, 1355 Oxford Street, PO Box 15000, Halifax, NS B3H 4R2, Canada.
E-mail address: penny.corkum@dal.ca

sleep.theclinics.com

Sleep problems in children with NDD, such as autism spectrum disorders (ASD) or ADHD, are even more prevalent than in TD children.[3] Between 50% and 95% of children with NDD meet criteria for a sleep disorder, with behavioral insomnia the most common sleep problem in this population.[4,5] These high rates are extremely concerning, given that poor sleep in children with NDD has been associated with impairments in many areas of functioning, based on caregiver ratings; for example, children with ASD and sleep problems have more severe symptoms of autism and more behavior problems.[6] Research has begun to establish that sleep problems add significantly to the morbidity of NDD and, as such, need to be adequately treated.

Behavioral insomnia is best conceptualized using a biopsychosocial framework. As highlighted in reviews by Reynolds and Malow[7] and Owens and colleagues,[8] there are many biologic and physiologic factors that may contribute to the development of insomnia in children with NDD, including

- Intrinsic abnormalities in neurobiological and circadian factors (eg, dysregulation of neurotransmitter systems having an impact on sleep and wakefulness and abnormal melatonin synthesis, timing, and regulation)
- Comorbid medical conditions (eg, epilepsy; gastrointestinal reflux disease; and physical concerns that may cause pain, discomfort, or sleep disruption, such as asthma and eczema)
- Comorbid psychiatric disorders (eg, anxiety and depression)
- Medication impact on sleep and wakefulness (eg, psychotropic medications, such as stimulants, and anticonvulsants)
- Other comorbid primary sleep disorders (eg, sleep-disordered breathing; parasomnias, such as sleep terrors, sleep walking, and confusional arousals; sleep-related movement disorders, such as restless legs syndrome and periodic limb movement disorder; and circadian rhythm disturbance, including delayed sleep phase disorder and irregular sleep-wake rhythm)

These are not the only factors, however, that should be targets of intervention. Rather, it is the behavioral factors—such as, inconsistent bedtime routines and poor sleep practices—that often set the stage for insomnia in TD children and also play a significant role in the cause of sleep problems in children with NDD.[9] In addition, some of the core symptoms of NDD (eg, hyperactivity, poor communication skills, and intellectual disability) may increase the risk of sleep problems and pose challenges for intervention. Common behavioral factors thought to contribute to insomnia in children with NDD include[7,9,10]

- Unhealthy sleep practices and patterns
- Hypersensitivity to environmental stimuli
- Hyperarousal/difficulty with self-regulation
- Repetitive thoughts/behaviors that interfere with settling at bedtime
- Inability to benefit from communicative/social cues about sleep

A substantial body of literature demonstrates the effectiveness of behavioral interventions in TD children with insomnia,[11] but there is little research in children with NDD. For example, a recent review of nonpharmacologic/behavioral sleep interventions for youth with chronic health conditions, including children with NDD, such as ASD and ADHD, identified 20 studies, the majority of which were single case studies or small group pre-/postcomparisons.[12] All studies demonstrated improvement in children's sleep, some studies found improved parental functioning, and none indicated any negative effects of using behavioral interventions to treat sleep problems in this population.

The purpose of this article is to describe behavioral insomnia and the impact of this common sleep problem in children with NDD and their families, with a focus on children with ASD and ADHD, 2 of the most common NDD, and to outline the process of assessing and treating behavioral insomnia using behavioral interventions that are modified to address the challenges of working with this population and to accommodate the needs of children with NDD.

SLEEP PROBLEMS IN ADHD

Children with ADHD have one of the highest rates of sleep problems of all children with mental health disorders. Prevalence estimates range between 50% and 95%, depending on how sleep problems are defined and measured.[4,13,14] ADHD has consistently been associated with sleep problems, and their presence was considered a diagnostic criterion for ADHD in an previous version of the *Diagnostic and Statistical Manual of Mental Disorders*.[14] Primary sleep problems, such as sleep-disordered breathing or narcolepsy, can certainly coexist in these children but are not the most common sleep problem in this population. Rather, the most common sleep complaints that parents of children with ADHD report are problems associated with behavioral insomnia (eg, resistance to bedtime and insufficient sleep).[14–17]

Research to date indicates that modifiable behavioral factors, which are amenable to treatment, play a significant role in the cause of sleep problems in this population.[16] These factors include child characteristics (eg, ADHD symptoms), family variables (eg, parent knowledge of healthy sleep practices, household routines, parental mental health, family composition, and family work and school schedules), and environmental factors (eg, child's bed/bedroom, access to television/computer, and noise level in house).

Children with ADHD and sleep problems have been found to have poorer outcomes than children with ADHD without sleep problems, including negative impact on behavior, cognitive functioning, and family functioning.[18,19] This is not surprising, given that sleep restriction in TD children can result in ADHD-like behaviors (eg, inattention and short-term memory problems).[20] Research has found that those children who have both ADHD and sleep problems experience increased behavioral problems[19,21] and poorer cognitive functioning, especially in executive functioning skills, such as working memory and attention.[22,23]

SLEEP PROBLEMS IN AUTISM SPECTRUM DISORDERS

Studies have also consistently documented high rates of sleep problems in children with ASD, with prevalence rates ranging from 53% to 78%.[24,25] The most common sleep problem in these children is insomnia (bedtime resistance, sleep-onset delay, and night or early morning waking).[24,25] The literature suggests that a majority of children with ASD have sleep difficulties, and the co-occurrence between the two is great enough that sleep difficulties may be characteristic of the ASD phenotype.[26,27] As discussed previously, there are several different neurophysiologic, medical, sleep, and psychiatric factors that can contribute to sleep problems in children with ASD.[7,28,29] Although it is important to address these factors whenever possible (eg, with medication adjustments and treatment of comorbid sleep disorders, such as obstructive sleep apnea), the focus of management of insomnia is most often on those modifiable contributory intrinsic and extrinsic behavioral factors, such as unhealthy sleep habits, inadequate parental limit setting, or hypersensitivity to environmental stimuli.[7,29]

Sleep problems in children with ASD are associated with deficits in daytime functioning and adaptive skills as well as emotional and behavioral problems. Such daytime behavioral problems may include increased rates of overactivity,[30] disruptive behaviors,[31] communication difficulties,[32] social problems, and difficulties with changes in routines.[32] These problems can affect or interfere with daytime learning and cognitive functioning.[6] Children identified as poor sleepers typically have a higher prevalence of behavioral problems than good sleepers and tend to have attentional and social interaction problems[33,34] and increased anxiety.[35] In younger children with ASD, poor sleep may be associated with language problems, aggression, hyperactivity, and poor adaptive functioning (eg, hygiene, toileting, and eating habits).[33,34]

Moreover, studies have suggested that as the severity of sleep problems increases, so does the severity of sequelae, such as behavioral problems and autism symptoms, sensory deficits, and gastrointestinal problems.[35–38] In particular, sleep-onset delay and sleep duration are positively correlated with autism symptoms and autism severity, with less sleep predicting overall autism symptom scores and social deficits.[6,38] Sleep-onset delay has been found the strongest predictor of communication deficits, stereotyped behavior, and autism severity.[38] Fewer hours of sleep per night and screaming during the night have been shown to predict stereotypic behavior.[6]

IMPACT OF CHILDREN'S SLEEP PROBLEMS ON PARENTS

Children's sleep problems have a direct impact on their parents and families. Levels of stress are typically higher in parents of children with NDD than in parents of children with TD children.[39–42] The literature suggests that parents of children with NDD report higher rates of sleep problems than do parents of TD children.[13,15] Therefore, it is not surprising that parents of children with NDD and sleep problems have increased parental stress.[43,44] A study examining sleep problems in children with ADHD revealed that primary caregivers of children with moderate to severe sleep problems were 3 times more likely to have elevated levels of stress and a higher risk of symptoms of depression and anxiety.[19] Likewise, children's poor sleep is a significant predictor of maternal stress for children with ASD.[45]

ASSESSMENT OF SLEEP PROBLEMS IN CHILDREN WITH NDD

Because of the high prevalence of sleep problems in this population, all children with NDD should be screened for sleep problems (**Fig. 1**).[29] Screening for sleep issues should be followed by identification of associated medical comorbidities that

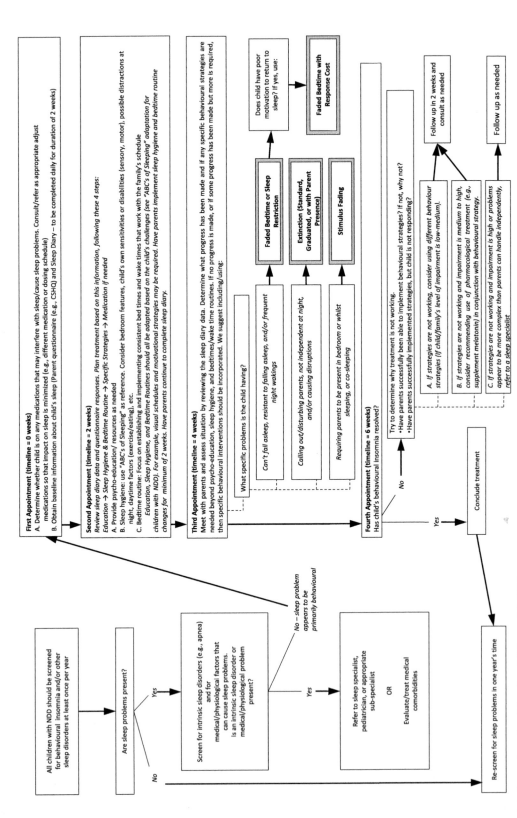

Fig. 1. Screening algorithm for children with NDD.

may affect children's sleep. A useful tool for this purpose is the Screening Checklist for Medical Comorbidities Associated with Sleep Problems,[7] developed by Reynolds and Malow from the Autism Treatment Network, which can be used by clinicians when interviewing families. Sleep problems in children with NDD can be identified and diagnosed using the same or modified assessment methods as for TD children (discussed later). See the treatment pathway in **Fig. 2** for guidelines on screening and assessment.

Children with NDD may be more sensitive to or less tolerant of certain types of assessment, in particular those that involve technological equipment. Therefore, specific adaptations may be required. **Table 1** highlights challenges that researchers and clinicians may face in using the most common objective and subjective measures of children's sleep to assess children with NDD and provides suggestions for how to address these challenges (see Hodge and colleagues[49] for a comprehensive review of methods of assessing sleep problems in children with ASD and Corkum and colleagues[10] for a comprehensive review of assessing sleep problems in children with ADHD). In general, a combination of objective measures (such as actigraphy) and subjective measures (such as parent-reported sleep diaries or questionnaires) is recommended.[10,49] For those readers less familiar with available sleep diagnostic tools, a brief description is provided later.

Objective Measures of Sleep

Polysomnography (PSG) is considered the gold standard for assessment of sleep.[49] PSG involves continuous electrophysiologic recordings of a child's overnight sleep and typically occurs in a sleep laboratory or hospital setting. PSG provides information on both the stages of sleep and the various physiologic parameters (cardiovascular, respiratory, and so forth) during sleep. It is primarily indicated to identify sleep-related breathing and movement disorders and may also be helpful in diagnosing parasomnias and nocturnal epilepsy in selected cases. Actigraphy, in conjunction with a sleep log, allows for the estimation of 24-hour sleep-wake patterns for extended periods of time

in the home setting. An actigraph is a watchlike device that captures and stores data regarding limb movements. Videosomnography involves the use of a portable, time-lapse recording system in a child's bedroom.[49,60] Observers review and code the recordings to determine sleep-wake states, total sleep time, and waking after sleep onset (WASO).

Subjective Measures of Sleep

Due to the frequency with which communication problems and intellectual disability occur in NDD, clinicians typically rely on parental report measures rather than child self-report measures.[49] Sleep diaries are used frequently and require daily reports from parents on children's sleep for the prior night. They are usually conducted over at least a 14-day period and should contain detailed information about bedtimes, waking time, sleep-onset time, presence of night waking, returning to sleep, and daytime napping.[62] Sleep diaries may be particularly useful in the assessment of behavioral insomnia in children with NDD; research shows that sleep diaries provide behavioral/environmental information about the presleep period as well as the morning period that may not be captured by objective measures of sleep but may be critical for understanding the contingencies giving rise to or maintaining sleep problems. For example, parents of children with ADHD report more problematic behaviors before bedtime, at bedtime, and in the morning compared with parents of TD children.[21]

Questionnaires are frequently recommended. The Children's Sleep Habits Questionnaire (CSHQ)[63] is a parent-report survey that was originally validated for children ages 4 through 10 years. It can be used to derive a total sleep disturbance score as well as 8 subscale scores (bedtime resistance, sleep-onset delay, sleep duration, sleep anxiety, night waking, parasomnias, sleep-disordered breathing, and daytime sleepiness). Recently, the CSHQ was found a clinically useful screening measure for children under 4 years of age as well,[64] including those with ASD.[65] The CSHQ is available free of charge from the authors who developed the measure (JOwens@childrensnational.org).

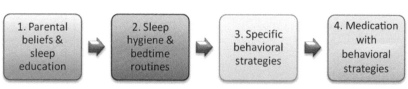

Fig. 2. Staged approach to the treatment of behavioral sleep problems. (*Adapted from* Weiss SK, Corkum P. Pediatric behavioural insomnia—"Good Night, Sleep Tight" for child and parent. Insomnia Rounds 2012;1(5):1–6.)

Table 1
Objective measures of sleep, challenges and suggestions for children with NDD

Measure	Challenges and Limitations	Advantages and Recommendations
PSG	Children with NDD who have sensory difficulties or sensitivities (eg, ASD) may find the procedure difficult to tolerate, because it requires application of sensors and an overnight stay in a sleep laboratory.[46] Research on children with ADHD specifically has shown that children with ADHD are more active during the night than control children, which may present problems during PSG, in which accurate assessment depends on the electrode sensors remaining connected during sleep.[47] There is also a possibility that children with ASD and ADHD may be more prone to difficulties adapting to sleeping in novel environments, the so-called first night effect. Research has demonstrated that TD children and children with ADHD showed differences between sleep at home and sleep at the sleep laboratory in certain sleep variables (eg, sleep duration) and as such caution must be taken when generalizing results from the sleep laboratory to home.[48]	The availability of a child-friendly sleep laboratory (eg, increased sleep technologist to child ratio [2:1 or 1:1]; sleeping accommodations for parents; adequate preparation, including availability of pre-PSG laboratory visits; and experienced staff) may mitigate the impact of the laboratory environment and diagnostic procedures. Research suggests that given the right accommodations and preparation, some children with NDD can adapt to a sleep laboratory. No similar research exists for children with ASD, but research exists in which PSG was successfully used with children with ASD (see Hodge and colleagues[49] for review). At-home PSG, which has been validated for use in clinical populations,[50] is an option for children with NDD.
Actigraphy	Although actigraphy is less invasive than PSG, there is concern that a sizable portion of children with NDD may not be able to tolerate wearing an actigraph due to sensory issues.[51–53] Actigraphy may also underestimate the frequency and duration of WASO in children with ASD, who frequently display contented sleeplessness (lying awake quietly[49,53]). There is also research showing that actigraphy is less accurate for children with ADHD (who have excessive movements) than for TD children.[54]	Previous research using actigraphy in children with NDD, such as ADHD, has been successful.[55,56] There is also evidence that actigraphy can be collected for children with ASD.[57] Preliminary research suggests that children who cannot tolerate wrist actigraphy may have the actigraph in a hidden pocket in their pajamas (eg, in the sleeve of the upper nondominant arm).[58,59]
Videosomnography	Children may become distracted by or focused on the camera, and cameras are relatively limited to focusing on one location only and cannot keep track of behavior that occurs away from this location.[49] For infants with NDD, the camera may be able to be placed very close to the crib. For older children with NDD, however, it may be necessary or recommended for the camera to be placed at a distance from the bed to be as unobtrusive as possible.[60,61] This distance, without the use of a telephoto lens, may make it difficult to score sleep states.	In a review of the literature on sleep assessment in children with ASD, Hodge and colleagues[49] suggested that because videosomnography is well tolerated and is relatively sensitive to WASO (which can be common in children with NDD), it may be a preferable way to objectively assess sleep in children with ASD, with or without actigraphy. To the authors' knowledge, only one study has explicitly examined the feasibility of time-lapse videosomnography in children with ASD and found it a successful technique.[61]

BEHAVIORAL MANAGEMENT OF SLEEP PROBLEMS IN CHILDREN

The most effective interventions for challenging behavior in children are those that use a behavioral approach. The symptoms of behavioral insomnia are no exception. Because behavioral insomnia takes place within the context of the relationship between a child and a parent, recommended treatment strategies are often based on parent-centered behavior management strategies. The underlying principle of the behavioral approach is that healthy sleep is a learned behavior.

Strategies for treating insomnia do not vary substantially between TD children and children with NDD. The underlying behavioral (eg, extinction and reinforcement) and psychophysiologic principles (eg, conditioning, circadian entrainment, and manipulation of sleep pressure/homeostatic processes) are consistent across populations. Considerations, however, such as the rate and scope of changes, external factors (eg, pain and mobility), and methods of implementation (eg, complexity of reward systems and use of visual cues and reminders), need to be incorporated in tailoring these interventions across populations and children.

A staged approach to the treatment of sleep problems is recommended,[66] with each stage representing a progressively more intensive intervention (**Fig. 2**).

Few recommendations for the course of treatment in this population have been developed, with the exception of the practice pathway created by Malow and colleagues[67] for children with ASD. Using a similar approach, the authors have developed a comprehensive treatment pathway for the screening of behavioral insomnia in children with NDD and the development and implementation of a behavioral treatment plan over 4 sessions (see appendix).

Parental Beliefs and Sleep Education

Ensuring that parents have accurate information about sleep and that their beliefs and sleep strategies are effective can be helpful both as a prevention strategy for the development of behavioral insomnia and as the first step in treatment.[68] **Box 1** highlights important aspects of addressing parental beliefs and providing psychoeducation about sleep.

Healthy Sleep Practices and Bedtime Routines

The development of good bedtime routines is one of the key components of any sleep intervention. The basic principles of healthy sleep habits are

---

Box 1
Parental beliefs and sleep education

- What parents know about children's sleep influences their beliefs and use of sleep strategies, which in turn has an impact on their children's sleep.
- Clinicians should
  - Discuss parents' knowledge and beliefs about sleep. Parents of children with NDD are especially likely to believe that their children's sleep problems are less modifiable and less responsive to treatment than are parents of TD children. It is important to ensure that they know sleep problems can often be successfully treated.
  - Emphasize to parents that poor sleep has negative consequences on children's daytime functioning and other areas of the family's life.
  - Identify which strategies parents have been using to deal with sleep problems and determine whether these strategies were appropriate and implemented appropriately.
  - Provide parents with accurate information about children's sleep and address any misconceptions, especially misconceptions related to
    - Causes of insomnia
    - Potential signs/symptoms of sleep problems
    - Consequences of poor sleep
    - Treatment of sleep problems
    - Modifiability of sleep scheduling
  - Emphasize to parents the importance of consistency and the establishment of a regular sleep schedule.

- Providing or creating an optimal sleep environment
- Sleep scheduling
- Sleep practice
- Physiologic sleep-promoting factors

Bessey and colleagues[69] published a useful and easy-to-remember mnemonic that captures the essence of healthy sleep practices, called "the ABCs of SLEEPING." For children with NDD, the ABCs of SLEEPING may require some modifications. Jan and colleagues[9] indicated that it may be more challenging to implement healthy sleep practices for children with NDD and that accommodations may need to be made with regard to environmental and sensory hypersensitivity as

Table 2
The ABCs of SLEEPING

Core Concept	Details and Recommendations	Modifications for NDD
A Age appropriate	It is important that children go to bed and wake up at times that ensure that they receive an age-appropriate amount of sleep. For children who have outgrown naps (which usually occurs during the preschool age period), napping during the day could be an indication that children are not getting sufficient quality and/or quantity of sleep at night.	Children with NDD often have intellectual disabilities as well as physical disabilities. It is important to consider these factors when determining what constitutes an age-appropriate amount of sleep. Generally, however, chronologic age is the best way to estimate how much sleep a child needs.
B Bedtimes	Having set bedtimes and wake times as well as routines in the evening and morning are key to good sleep. It is recommended that bedtimes be no later than 9:00 PM across childhood.[70]	When setting bedtimes and wake times for children with NDD, clinicians and parents must consider the timing of medication (eg, stimulant medication) and impact on sleep. One of the best ways to help children with NDD (especially those who are nonverbal or intellectually delayed or easily distracted) stick to routines is by using visual schedules, or visual, picture-based depictions of routines. This may take the form of a picture schedule or picture chart.
C Consistency	Bedtimes and wake times must be consistent, even on weekends (ie, no more than 30–60 min difference between weekday and weekend bedtimes and wake times).[71,72]	For children with NDD, ensuring that bedtimes and wake times are consistent is critically important because they may have more difficulty regulating their behavior and settling at night.
S Schedule and routines	Children's schedules in general are important—in addition to having routines at bedtime and wake time, it is also important that they have consistency throughout their day, including the timing of homework, extracurricular activities, etc.	Children with NDD may need to take extra time for transitions between activity and sleep and may require increased verbal prompts and reminders. Although children with NDD typically respond well to routines, sometimes they can become overly fixated on routines and refuse to go to sleep unless routines are followed very specifically (eg, as with ASD). Introducing a small amount of variability into the bedtime routine each night (eg, reading a different book or wearing different pajamas each night) may help prevent this and promote flexibility.[73]
L Location	It is important that a child's location for sleep includes a comfortable bed; the room is quiet, dark, and cool; and the location should be consistent and familiar. Also, children's bedrooms should be used only for sleeping—children should not be sent to their bedroom for a time out. Their bedroom also should not be too exciting or distracting and should be conducive to relaxation.	Children with NDD may have motor disabilities, sensory sensitivities, and hypersensitivity to environmental stimuli, all of which can influence how to arrange the bedroom (eg, lighting, physical comfort of bed, placement of bed, and temperature). Therefore, it is important to 1. Reduce opportunities for distractions in the bedroom 2. Consider any sensory issues, pain, or discomfort that may affect sleeping

E	No Electronics in the bedroom or before bed	The use of electronics, including both the timing of use and the location, should also be considered—children should not be using stimulating electronic devices (iPods, cell phones, laptops, etc.) too close to bedtime (most commonly defined as 1 h prior to going to bed[74]), and it is recommended that these items not be placed in the bedroom.	Many children with NDD enjoy electronics, such as video or computer games or television. As previously indicated, parents should reduce opportunities for distractions in the bedroom by removing such devices.
E	Exercise and diet	Exercise and diet are both important factors that should be considered when evaluating sleep practices—physical activity during the day is important to healthy sleep but should not be undertaken too close to bedtime (defined in the literature as anywhere from 1 h to 4 h prior to bedtime[75]). Diet concerns around sleep include caffeine consumption—children should limit or totally eliminate intake of caffeinated foods or beverages—as well as the timing of meals. Children should not be going to bed hungry, but they also should not be consuming a large meal right before bedtime.	Ensuring that children with NDD get sufficient opportunities for exercise is critical, in particular children who prefer sedentary activities. Physical activity, however, should not take place too close to bedtime. Heavy meals should be avoided at bedtime.[9]
P	Positivity and relaxation	Positivity surrounding sleep is also an important aspect of sleep practices. Parents should have a positive attitude toward sleep and the bedtime/wake time routine, and the atmosphere in the house should be positive to be conducive to creating a positive mood in children. It is important that this positive mood is relaxing and calming, rather than fun and exciting—children should be winding down before bedtime. Also, doing frustrating activities right before bed (eg, math problems for a child who struggles with math) is not recommended, because this may interfere with children's ability to fall asleep.	Positive reinforcement from parents is important for children with NDD, especially during potentially stressful times, such as the bedtime routine. Children with NDD may require additional assistance with unwinding or reducing stimulation before bed. Bedtime activities should be calming and simple. Activities that involve new or unexpected events (which can be frustrating or challenging), excessive noise, or vigorous exercise may be overstimulating and either make the bedtime routine too stimulating or wind children up too much to relax to sleep.[9]
I	Independence when falling asleep	Independence is also important. Once children reach an age where they are capable of settling into sleep without their parents, independence when falling asleep should be encouraged to discourage dependence on someone else to fall asleep. For children, independence means no calling out and no getting out of bed, and for parents, no responding to children calling out and returning children to their room if they do get out of bed.	Although children with NDD may sometimes require help or supervision from their parents or caregivers in other areas of daily functioning, sleep is an aspect of their lives where developing independence is critical. For children with NDD, sleep independence means staying in bed and not calling out, and for their parents, this means unbroken and peaceful sleep.
N	Needs met during the day	Finally, the needs of children should be met throughout the day. This refers to both children's emotional needs (love, support, hugs, etc.) and basic physiologic needs (thirst, hunger, etc.).	Given that there are often many demands on parents during the day, it is often harder to meet all of a child's needs in the daytime. Children with NDD work hard to regulate themselves and it is important for parents to recognize this and provide love and support. Having positive time with parents should be a feature of both daytime and bedtime routines.
G	All of the above equals a Great sleep!		

From Bessey M, Coulombe JA, Corkum P. Sleep hygiene in children with AD/HD: findings and recommendations. ADHD Rep 2013;21(3):1–7.

Table 3
Behavioral strategies and adaptations for children with NDD

Strategy	Primary Use	Adaptation for Children with NDD	Research Examples
Sleep scheduling	Sleep scheduling: this is the essence of healthy sleep practices and behavioral treatment. It is vital to schedule regular, age-appropriate sleep and wake times that allow children the opportunity to have adequate sleep.	Children with NDD may require increased support as their parents implement new routines and bedtimes in the form of • Increased transitional warnings ("10 more minutes until it's time to get ready for bed...5 more minutes...2 more minutes," etc.) • Additional prompts and reminders about bedtimes • Use of visual supports and schedules	• Moon et al, 2011 (3 children with ASD, age 8–9 y, integrated with FBRC)[78] • Mullane and Corkum, 2006 (3 children with ADHD, age 8–9 y, integrated with FBRC)[56]
Extinction	Standard (unmodified) extinction: a child is put to bed while awake and left alone until he or she falls asleep. Any night wakings are ignored by parents. A child learns to self-soothe once he or she realizes that crying at night or calling for parents does not result in getting parental attention. Graduated extinction: like standard extinction, a child is put to bed while awake and left to fall asleep. In this case, however, the parents ignore the child's negative behaviors (eg, crying, night waking, and calling out) for a specified amount of time before they check in on	Child frequently calls out at night, disturbs parents, and causes disruptions. Child is not independent at night. As described directly above. Graduated extinction/ extinction with parent presences may be more appealing options for parents who are reluctant to	Parents should be aware that using an extinction technique may result in a temporary increase in negative behaviors (called an extinction burst), which can be distressing and especially problematic in children with self-injurious behavior. It is important for clinicians to educate parents about extinction bursts and provide support as the extinction technique is implemented.[76] If children with NDD have sensory, motor, or other	• Weiskop et al, 2005 (5 children with ASD + 5 children with fragile X syndrome, ages 3–7 y old, problems with night wakings)[79] • Wolf et al, 1964 (in-patient child with ASD, violent tantrums associated with night waking)[80] • Durand et al, 1996 (2 children with ASD, bedtime disturbances, and problems initiating sleep)[81] • Moore, 2004 (1 child with ASD, cosleeping, problems initiating sleep)[82]

the child. Gradually, the parent increases the amount of time between hearing crying and responding (coming to check on the child). Parents provide reassurance through their presence but only for short duration and with minimal interaction. Variation: extinction with parent presence. The child is put to bed while awake. The parent remains in the room until he or she falls asleep, acting as a reassurance. The parent, however, provides little interaction or attention for crying, etc. The parent's presence is the child's comfort.	leave their child in distress or let them "cry it out."	disabilities, it may be important not to leave them entirely alone—parents may want to unobtrusively check in by leaving a door open or keep track of their child using baby monitors, video camera, etc. With any extinction technique, positive reinforcement of desired behaviors is especially helpful. Using strategies, such as a token economy (described later), may be a good way to do this. If children have severe behavioral problems in addition to sleep problems (eg, disruptive/ externalizing/destructive behaviors), extinction may not be the best option for them.	• Mullane & Corkum, 2006 (2 children with ADHD + primary insomnia + cosleeping —use of systematic ignoring)[56]
Extinction— stimulus fading: the goal of stimulus fading is to reduce cosleeping with parents, and the main focus is to gradually reduce and then eliminate a parent's presence from the child's room. For example, on night 1, the parent might sleep on mattress beside the child's bed, and on successive nights, the mattress is moved farther away from the bed until it is out of the room.	Child requires parents to be present in bedroom or while sleeping. Child cosleeps with parents.		• Howlin, 1984 (case study of 5 y old with ASD with night wakings and cosleeping)[83] • Reed et al, 2009 (21 children with ASD, multicomponent intervention, including stimulus fading, extinction, and group parent education workshop)[84]

(continued on next page)

Table 3
(continued)

	Strategy	Primary Use	Adaptation for Children with NDD	Research Examples
Faded bedtime/ sleep restriction	Faded bedtime: parents identify a target bedtime or goal (the time at which they want their child to fall asleep). They then proceed to delay or fade the actual bedtime over a period of days or weeks, moving it closer to the target bedtime. The goal is for the child to develop a positive association between being in bed and falling asleep quickly—for children to learn to fall asleep when they are tired. Bedtimes can gradually be moved earlier. Typically, the child is awakened at the same time each morning and is not allowed to sleep outside of the set sleep times. This technique can be used in conjunction with sleep restriction. FBRC: this technique takes the faded bedtime strategy (as described directly above) and adds a response cost component, which is generally a desired or enjoyable, but not overly stimulating, activity. A sample FBRC plan might be 1. Putting child to bed at a specific time. If child does not fall asleep within 20 min, he or she is removed from bed and must spend 20 min engaging in a quiet, nonrewarding activity. 2. After the 20-min activity, the child is placed back to bed. If he or she is unable to fall asleep within 20 min, he or she again is removed from bed for 20 min.	Faded bedtime techniques are most useful for children who have problems initiating and/or maintaining sleep. They can also be used to deal with bedtime disturbances, for example, when children are reluctant to go to bed, stay in bed, or stay awake for long periods of time after being put into bed. Adding a response cost component may be especially helpful if a child has poor motivation to return to sleep after waking up. Including a sleep restriction component may be helpful, especially if it is believed that less sleep may help the child become sleepier and therefore fall asleep faster. Positive bedtime routines can be used additionally to reduce bedtime disturbances and night waking.	When using faded bedtime or sleep restriction techniques, it may be helpful to provide a child with positive reinforcers. Parents should be aware that reinforcers can be idiosyncratic and may not always work. It can be difficult to find appropriately motivating positive reinforcers for children with NDD (especially those with ASD). Activity-based reinforcers may be most effective. It is important to ensure that activity-based reinforcers are • Not too rewarding • Not overly stimulating • Not electronics-based (eg, no TV, video games, or smartphone) Equally important is to ensure that response cost activities are • Relatively boring and relaxing • Not dependent on parent presence Children with NDD may have a tendency to become overaroused (ADHD) or overly fixated on an activity (ASD). For example, children with ASD tend to find their own special interests or preoccupations	• DeLeon et al, 2004 (case study of 4-year-old boy with ASD and developmental delay, and self-injurious behavior associated with night waking)[85] • Moon et al, 2011 (3 children with ASD between ages 5 and 9 y with difficulty initiating sleep)[78] • Piazza et al, 1997 (3 children with ASD between ages 5 and 9 y on inpatient ward with difficulty initiating sleep + severe behavior problems)[86] • Mullane & Corkum, 2006 (3 children with ADHD + primary insomnia, bedtime resistance)[56]

3. This procedure is repeated until the child is able to fall asleep within 20 min of being placed back in bed.
4. Once a child is able to fall asleep within 20 min at a specific bedtime for a few consecutive nights, the bedtime is moved earlier (in 15–30-min increments) until the target bedtime is achieved.

This technique can be used in conjunction with sleep restriction.

Sleep restriction: this technique involves fading bedtime and is similar to FBRC. It is based, however, on sleep duration, instead of bedtime. Parents limit the time that a child spends in bed to 90% of the child's baseline total sleep duration. This restricts the total amount of time the child spends awake in bed. The parents and clinician determine a target in terms of how much they would like sleep disturbances to decrease; if the child achieves this target, then the bedtime is faded 15 min earlier each week. Should the child remain awake in bed, the response cost technique is used. Sleep restriction techniques should be used in conjunction with positive bedtime routines, to decrease night waking and bedtime disturbances.[9]

most rewarding and can be resistant to the interruption of these activities to go to bed.[78]

It is important for parents to know that sleep restriction can result in some increased difficulty implementing bedtime routines due to problematic behavior (eg, Christodulu and Durand, 2004).[87]

- Christodulu & Durand, 2004 (4 y old with ASD, bedtime disturbance, and night waking)[87]
- Durand et al, 2004 (4 y old with ASD, cosleeping, bedtime disturbance, and night waking)[88]
- Gruber et al, 2011 (1 h of nightly sleep restriction on 11 children with ADHD, ages 7–11 y)[22]

(continued on next page)

Table 3
(continued)

Strategy	Primary Use	Adaptation for Children with NDD	Research Examples
Cognitive strategies	Cognitive strategies: cognitive strategies can be used to help both children and parents. For example, cognitive strategies can address unhelpful or unproductive beliefs about sleep (eg, the child cannot change his/her sleep difficulty). They can also include coping strategies, such as learning relaxation skills (eg, deep abdominal breathing). Cognitive strategies can also help children learn how to handle anxiety, which can cause sleep problems. Cognitive behavior therapy for sleep problems can include a combination of cognitive therapies, relaxation training, stimulus control therapy, and sleep restriction.[89]	May be helpful for children who have co-occurring anxiety, especially anxiety about sleep. Can also be useful to help prepare parents for treatment and to stop and deal with negative thoughts about sleep problems. Cognitive interventions differ based on the age of the child having sleep problems. For infants and toddlers, cognitive strategies usually focus on changing parental cognitions and behaviors to affect a child's sleep. For preschool and school-age children, cognitive strategies can target age-specific developmental issues (eg, nighttime fears or bedtime refusal) and a clinician can work with the child directly. Likewise, for adolescents, cognitive behavior therapy for insomnia may be helpful in addressing the stress associated with sleep problems and how to cope with other areas of worry.[90]	Working with children: children with NDD often have comorbid anxiety, but anxiety might not look like anxiety—it may look like acting out or disruptive behavior. Cognitive strategies and teaching relaxation skills do not cure anxiety but can help children manage their feelings and gain some control. Techniques, such as guided imagery, can help reduce anxiety and psychological arousal at bedtime.[10] Working with the parent(s): it is important to help parents maintain their motivation for implementing treatment, especially when they are sleep-deprived. It may be helpful to focus with parents on what their in-the-moment thoughts are (eg, when a child is crying at night), especially if they are having trouble sticking to treatment guidelines (eg, not responding to child crying). Furthermore, clinicians may need to reassure parents that sleep problems can be treated, because parents of children with NDD may have specific	• Malow et al, 2014 (parent-based sleep education, group and individual therapy—for parents of 80 children with ASD ages 2–10 y old)[93]

163

	Cognitive strategies may be helpful in eliminating cosleeping (especially when cosleeping is due to anxiety or nighttime fears).	beliefs about sleep problems in their children.[91] Research has shown that parental behaviors during bedtime and the night are influenced by their cognitions and emotions[90] and that sleep problems affect family functioning and parenting sensitivity.[92]	
Reward and reinforce-ment programs	Reward and reinforcement programs: using reward and reinforcement programs can help motivate children, increase wanted behaviors (eg, sleeping soundly, not disturbing parents) and decrease unwanted behaviors (eg, crying or calling out). One useful technique that can be used in conjunction with the behavior strategies is the token economy. Children earn tokens (such as stickers), which can be traded or cashed in for larger prizes once a parent-decided number of tokens has been earned. Opportunities to earn tokens may include • Completing their bedtime routines • Trying to fall asleep quietly and • Staying in bed without calling out to parents	Reward and reinforcement programs can be used in conjunction with any of these techniques in order to increase wanted behaviors and decrease unwanted behaviors. Rewards/reinforcement may be particularly indicated in cases where a child has problematic behaviors or bedtime disturbances. Helpful NDD modifications: • Having a visual reminder of what the expectations are for a token economy • Placing a sticker chart where children can see it may increase motivation • Stickers or tokens may need to be cashed in more often to maintain a child's motivation • Token economies may not work as well for children with poor verbal skills	• Weiskop et al, 2005 (children with ASD, 3–7 y old; sticker charts, visual representations of bedtime routines + extinction)[79]

well as the potential for overadherence to routines. **Table 2** lists the original ABCs in the left column, with suggested modifications for children with NDD in the right column.

Specific Behavioral Strategies

Behavioral interventions are based on applied behavioral analysis and can include techniques, such as token economies, extinction, graduated extinction, fading, and response cost. There has been little research on which behavioral strategies for sleep problems work for children with NDD.[76] A recent review of treatment strategies for complex behavioral insomnia in children with NDD endorsed the use of these behavioral interventions as a first-line treatment of children with ASD, followed by supplements, such as oral melatonin or other medications, should problems remain (discussed below in the next section). Above all, the review emphasized that the foundation of insomnia therapy in NDD is caregivers as agents for change of problematic sleep behaviors.[77]

Several specific behavioral interventions have been found effective in reducing sleep problems in TD children in several studies, and there is a growing body of research demonstrating that these interventions can be extended to children with NDD. **Table 3** highlights these interventions, with suggestions for adapting them to children with NDD.

Medication as an Adjunct to Behavioral Therapy

Although the topic of use of sedative/hypnotic medication in children with NDD is beyond the scope of this review, medication may be considered as an adjunct to behavioral management of insomnia in selected cases. In particular, several studies have suggested that use of synthetic melatonin either as a chronobiotic (small dose 4–7 hours before sleep onset) or mild hypnotic (larger dose just before bedtime) may be effective in reducing sleep-onset delay in children with ADHD and ASD. For a systematic review of melatonin use in children with neurodevelopmental disabilities, see Phillips and Appleton[94]; for a review of melatonin use in children with ASD, see Rossingnol and Frye[95] or Guénolé and colleagues[96]; and for a review of melatonin use in children with ADHD, see Bendz and Scates[97] or Hoebert and colleagues.[98] Medication should never be the first or sole treatment choice and a medication trial (including over-the-counter drugs) should be initiated only after consultation with a health care professional (eg, pediatrician or sleep specialist). For more information on how medications for sleep disorders in

---

Box 2
Online resources for clinicians and parents

- Sleep Tool Kit (Parent Booklet), from Autism Speaks
  - http://www.autismspeaks.org/science/resources-programs/autism-treatment-network/tools-you-can-use/sleep-tool-kit
- Children's Sleep Network
  - http://www.childrenssleepnetwork.org/WP/
- Chronic Care for Sleep: Web-based help for sleep problems in children with neurodevelopmental conditions
  - http://www.chroniccare4sleep.org/About.html
- Better Nights, Better Days: a sleep study for parents with children who have sleeping problems
  - http://betternightsbetterdays.ca/
- Dalhousie Child Clinical and School Psychology Lab: learning, attention, behavior, sleep
  - http://myweb.dal.ca/pvcorkum/

NDD can be used in conjunction with behavioral interventions, see review by Ahmareen and colleagues[99] or Hollway and Aman.[100] For a thorough review of pharmacology for sleep problems in ASD, see Johnson and Malow,[101] and for a review of pharmacotherapy for sleep problems in ADHD, see Corkum and colleagues[10] and Barrett and colleagues[102] (**Box 2**).

SUMMARY

Sleep problems represent a real and troubling aspect of the lives of many children with NDD. As with TD children, the most common sleep problem among children with NDD is behavioral insomnia. Prevalence rates of sleep problems in general range between 50% and 95% for children with NDD. Given that poor sleep in children with NDD has been associated with impairments in daytime functioning, decreased quality of life for the children, increased NDD symptoms and morbidity, and negative effects on caregivers' health and parenting abilities, these high rates are concerning and underscore the need for appropriate screening, diagnostic evaluation, and management. Behavioral interventions have considerable empiric support and should be recommended as first-line treatment of sleep problems in this population. Additional research is needed to establish the effectiveness of specific behavioral strategies, including psycho-education, healthy sleep practices, and techniques, such as faded bedtime with response cost (FBRC) or extinction, for treating behavioral insomnia in children with NDD.

REFERENCES

1. Owens J. Classification and epidemiology of childhood sleep disorders. Sleep Med Clin 2007;2(3): 353–61.

2. Moore M, Meltzer LJ, Mindell JA. Bedtime problems and night wakings in children. Sleep Med Clin 2007;2(3):377–85.

3. Ivanenko A, Gururaj BR. Classification and epidemiology of sleep disorders. Child Adolesc Psychiatr Clin N Am 2009;18(4):839–48.

4. Corkum P, Tannock R, Moldofsky H. Sleep disturbances in children with attention-deficit/hyperactivity disorder. J Am Acad Child Psychiatry 1998;37(6):637–46.

5. Polimeni MA, Richdale AL, Francis AJ. A survey of sleep problems in autism, asperger's disorder and typically developing children. J Intellect Disabil Res 2005;49(4):260–8.

6. Schreck KA, Mulick JA, Smith AF. Sleep problems as possible predictors of intensified symptoms of autism. Res Dev Disabil 2004;25(1):57–66.

7. Reynolds AM, Malow B. Sleep and autism spectrum disorders. Pediatr Clin North Am 2011;58: 685–98.

8. Owens J, Gruber R, Brown T, et al. Future research directions in sleep and ADHD: report of a consensus working group. J Atten Disord 2013; 17(7):550–64.

9. Jan JE, Owens JA, Weiss MD, et al. Sleep hygiene for children with neurodevelopmental disabilities. Pediatrics 2008;122(6):1343–50.

10. Corkum P, Davidson F, MacPherson M. A framework for the assessment and treatment of sleep problems in children with attention-deficit/hyperactivity disorder. Pediatr Clin North Am 2011;58:667–83.

11. Mindell JA, Kuhn B, Lewin DS, et al. Behavioral treatment of bedtime problems and night wakings in infants and young children. Sleep 2006;29(10): 1263–76.

12. Brown CA, Kuo M, Phillips L, et al. Non-pharmacological sleep interventions for youth with chronic health conditions: a critical review of the methodological quality of the evidence. Disabil Rehabil 2013;35(15):1221–55.

13. Cortese S, Faraone SV, Konofal E, et al. Sleep in children with attention-deficit/hyperactivity disorder: meta-analysis of subjective and objective studies. J Am Acad Child Psychiatry 2009;48(9): 894–908.

14. Owens JA. The ADHD and sleep conundrum: a review. J Dev Behav Pediatr 2005;26(4):312–22.

15. Corkum P, Moldofsky H, Hogg-Johnson S, et al. Sleep problems in children with attention-deficit/hyperactivity disorder: impact of subtype, comorbidity, and stimulant medication. J Am Acad Child Psychiatry 1999;38(10):1285–93.

16. Corkum P, Coulombe JA. Sleep in the context of AD/HD: a review of reviews to determine implications for research and clinical practice. In: Montgomery-Downs H, Wolfson AR, editors. The Oxford handbook of infant, child, and adolescent sleep: development and problems. New York: Oxford University Press; 2013. p. 495–514.

17. Meltzer LJ, Mindell JA. Sleep and sleep disorders in children and adolescents. Psychiatr Clin North Am 2006;29(4):1059–76.

18. Owens JA, Maxim R, Nobile C, et al. Parental and self-report of sleep in children with attention-deficit/hyperactivity disorder. Arch Pediatr Adolesc Med 2000;154:549–55.

19. Sung V, Hiscock H, Sciberras E, et al. Sleep problems in children with attention-deficit/hyperactivity disorder: prevalence and the effect on the child and family. Arch Pediatr Adolesc Med 2008;162: 336–42.

20. Vriend JL, Davidson FD, Corkum PV, et al. Manipulating sleep duration alters emotional functioning and cognitive performance in children. J Pediatr Psychol 2013;38(10):1058–69.

21. Owens J, Sangal RB, Sutton VK, et al. Subjective and objective measures of sleep in children with attention-deficit/hyperactivity disorder. Sleep Med 2009;10(4):446–56.

22. Gruber R, Wiebe S, Montecalvo L, et al. Impact of sleep restriction on neurobehavioral functioning of children with attention deficit hyperactivity disorder. Sleep 2011;34(3):315–23.

23. Moreau V, Rouleau N, Morin CM. Sleep, attention, and executive functioning in children with attention-deficit/hyperactivity disorder. Arch Clin Neuropsychol 2013;28:692–9.

24. Couturier JL, Speechley KN, Steele M, et al. Parental perception of sleep problems in children of normal intelligence with pervasive developmental disorders: prevalence, severity, and pattern. J Am Acad Child Psychiatry 2005;44(8): 815–22.

25. Krakowiak P, Goodlin-Jones B, Hertz-Picciotto I, et al. Sleep problems in children with autism spectrum disorders, developmental delays, and typical development: a population-based study. J Sleep Res 2008;17(2):197–206.

26. Limoges É, Bolduc C, Berthiaume C, et al. Relationship between poor sleep and daytime cognitive performance in young adults with autism. Res Dev Disabil 2013;34(4):1322–35.

27. Richdale AL, Prior MR. The sleep/wake rhythm in children with autism. Eur Child Adolesc Psychiatry 1995;4(3):175–86.

28. Johnson KP, Giannotti F, Cortesi F. Sleep patterns in autism spectrum disorders. Child Adolesc Psychiatr Clin N Am 2009;18(4):917–28.

29. Johnson KP, Malow B. Sleep in children with autism spectrum disorders. Curr Treat Options Neurol 2008;10:350–9.

30. Hoshino Y, Watanabe H, Yashima Y, et al. An investigation on sleep disturbance of autistic children. Folia Psychiatr Neurol Jpn 1984;38:45–52.

31. Patzold LM, Richdale AL, Tonge BJ. An investigation into sleep characteristics of children with autism and asperger's disorder. J Paediatr Child Health 1998;34:528–33.

32. Segawa M, Katoh M, Katoh J, et al. Early modulation of sleep parameters and its importance in later behavior. Brain Dysfunct 1992;5(3–4):211–23.

33. Goldman SE, McGrew S, Johnson KP, et al. Sleep is associated with problem behaviors in children and adolescents with autism spectrum disorders. Res Autism Spectr Disord 2011;5(3):1223–9.

34. Taylor MA, Schreck KA, Mulick JA. Sleep disruption as a correlate to cognitive and adaptive behavior problems in autism spectrum disorders. Res Dev Disabil 2012;33(5):1408–17.

35. Sikora DM, Johnson K, Clemons T, et al. The relationship between sleep problems and daytime behavior in children of different ages with autism spectrum disorders. Pediatrics 2012;130(Suppl 2):S83–90.

36. Hollway JA, Aman MG, Butter E. Correlates and risk markers for sleep disturbance in participants of the autism treatment network. J Autism Dev Disord 2013;43(12):2830–43.

37. Mayes SD, Calhoun SL. Variables related to sleep problems in children with autism. Res Autism Spectr Disord 2009;3(4):931–41.

38. Tudor ME, Hoffman CD, Sweeney DP. Children with autism: sleep problems and symptom severity. Focus Autism Other Dev Stud 2012; 27(4):254–62.

39. Abbeduto L, Seltzer MM, Shattuck P, et al. Psychological well-being and coping in mothers of youths with autism, down syndrome, or fragile X syndrome. Am J Ment Retard 2004;109(3):237–54.

40. Higgins DJ, Bailey SR, Pearce JC. Factors associated with functioning style and coping strategies of families with a child with an autism spectrum disorder. Autism 2005;9(2):125–37.

41. Perry A. A model of stress in families of children with developmental disabilities: clinical and research applications. J Dev Disabl 2005;11:1–16.

42. Perry A, Harris K, Minnes P. Family environments and family harmony: an exploration across severity, age, and type of DD. J Dev Disabl 2005;11:17–30.

43. Doo S, Wing YK. Sleep problems of children with pervasive developmental disorders: correlation with parental stress. Dev Med Child Neurol 2006; 48(8):650–5.

44. Noble GS, O'Laughlin L, Brubaker B. Attention deficit hyperactivity disorder and sleep disturbances: consideration of parental influence. Behav Sleep Med 2012;10:41–53.

45. Hoffman CD, Sweeney DP, Hodge D, et al. Parenting stress and closeness: mothers of typically developing children and mothers of children with autism. Focus Autism Other Dev Stud 2009;24(3): 178–87.

46. Arbelle S, Ben-Zion I. Sleep problems in autism. In: Schopler E, Yirmiya N, Shulman C, et al, editors. The research basis for autism intervention. New York: Kluwer Academic/Plenum Publishers; 2001. p. 219–27.

47. Konofal E, Lecendreux M, Bouvard MP, et al. High levels of nocturnal activity in children with attention-deficit hyperactivity disorder: a video analysis. Psychiatry Clin Neurosci 2001;55(2): 97–103.

48. Bessey M, Richards J, Corkum P. Sleep lab adaptation in children with attention-deficit/hyperactivity disorder and typically developing children. Sleep Disord 2013;2013:698957. Available at: http://www.hindawi.com/journals/sd/2013/698957/abs/. Accessed December 10, 2013.

49. Hodge D, Parnell AM, Hoffman CD, et al. Methods for assessing sleep in children with autism spectrum disorders: a review. Res Autism Spectr Disord 2012;6(4):1337–44.

50. Santos-Silva R, Sartori DE, Truksinas V, et al. Validation of a portable monitoring system for the diagnosis of obstructive sleep apnea syndrome. Sleep 2009;32(5):629–36.

51. Hering E, Epstein R, Elroy S, et al. Sleep patterns in autistic children. J Autism Dev Disord 1999;29(2): 143–7.

52. Øyane NM, Bjorvatn B. Sleep disturbances in adolescents and young adults with autism and asperger syndrome. Autism 2005;9(1):83–94.

53. Wiggs L, Stores G. Sleep patterns and sleep disorders in children with autistic spectrum disorders: insights using parent report and actigraphy. Dev Med Child Neurol 2004;46(6):372–80.

54. Waldon J, Gendron M, Corkum P. Concordance of actigraphy and polysomnography in school-aged children with attention-deficit/hyperactivity disorder and their typically developing peers. Poster session presented at: 73rd Annual Canadian Psychological Association Convention. Halifax, Nova Scotia (Canada), June 14–16, 2012.

55. Corkum P, Panton R, Ironside S, et al. Acute impact of immediate release methylphenidate administered three times a day on sleep in children with

attention-deficit/hyperactivity disorder. J Pediatr Psychol 2008;33(4):368–79.

56. Mullane J, Corkum P. Case series: evaluation of a behavioral sleep intervention for three children with attention-Deficit/Hyperactivity disorder and dyssomnia. J Atten Disord 2006;10(2):217–27.

57. Cortesi F, Giannotti F, Sebestiani T, et al. Controlled-release melatonin, singly and combined with cognitive behavioural therapy, for persistent insomnia in children with autism spectrum disorders: a randomized placebo-controlled trial. J Sleep Res 2012;21(6):700–9.

58. Adkins KW, Goldman SE, Fawkes D, et al. A pilot study of shoulder placement for actigraphy in children. Behav Sleep Med 2012;10(2):138–47.

59. Souders MC, Mason TB, Valladares O, et al. Sleep behaviors and sleep quality in children with autism spectrum disorders. Sleep 2009;32(12):1566–78.

60. Anders TF, Sostek AM. The use of time lapse video recording of sleep-wake behavior in human infants. Psychophysiology 1976;13(2):155–8.

61. Honomichl RD, Goodlin-Jones B, Burnham MM, et al. Secretin and sleep in children with autism. Child Psychiatry Hum Dev 2002;33(2):107–23.

62. Stores G. Sleep-wake function in children with neurodevelopmental and psychiatric disorders. Semin Pediatr Neurol 2001;8(4):188–97.

63. Owens JA, Spirito A, McGuinn M. The children's sleep habits questionnaire (CSHQ): psychometric properties of a survey instrument for school-aged children. Sleep 2000;23(8):1–9.

64. Owens JA, Fernando S, McGuinn M. Sleep disturbance and injury risk in young children. Behav Sleep Med 2005;3(1):18–31.

65. Goodlin-Jones B, Sitnick SL, Tang K, et al. The children's sleep habits questionnaire in toddlers and preschool children. J Dev Behav Pediatr 2008; 29(2):82–8.

66. Reid GJ, Hong RY, Wade TJ. The relation between common sleep problems and emotional and behavioral problems among 2- and 3-year-olds in the context of known risk factors for psychopathology. J Sleep Res 2009;18(1):49–59.

67. Malow BA, Byars K, Johnson K, et al. A practice pathway for the identification, evaluation, and management of insomnia in children and adoelscents with autism spectrum disorders. Pediatrics 2012; 130(Suppl 2):S106–24.

68. Weiss SK, Corkum P. Pediatric behavioral insomnia—"Good Night, Sleep Tight" for child and parent. Insomnia Rounds 2012;1(5):1–6. Available at: www.insomniarounds.ca.

69. Bessey M, Coulombe JA, Corkum P. Sleep hygiene in children with AD/HD: findings and recommendations. ADHD Rep 2013;21(3):1–7.

70. Mindell JA, Meltzer LJ, Carskadon MA, et al. Developmental aspects of sleep hygiene: findings from the 2004 national sleep foundation sleep in America poll. Sleep Med 2009;10(7):771–9.

71. Biggs SN, Lushington K, van den Heuvel CJ, et al. Inconsistent sleep schedules and daytime behavioral difficulties in school-aged children. Sleep Med 2011;12(8):780–6.

72. Gruber R, Cassoff J, Knauper B. Sleep health education in pediatric community settings: rationale and practical suggestions for incorporating healthy sleep education into pediatric practice. Pediatr Clin North Am 2011;58(3):735–54.

73. Kodak T, Piazza CC. Assessment and behavioral treatment of feeding and sleeping disorders in children with autism spectrum disorders. Child Adolesc Psychiatr Clin N Am 2008;17(4): 887–905.

74. LeBourgeois M, Giannotti F, Cortesi F, et al. The relationship between reported sleep quality and sleep hygiene in Italian and American adolescents. Pediatrics 2005;115:257–65.

75. Harvey AG. Sleep hygiene and sleep-onset insomnia. J Nerv Ment Dis 2000;188(1):53–5.

76. Vriend JL, Corkum PV, Moon EC, et al. Behavioral interventions for sleep problems in children with autism spectrum disorders: current findings and future directions. J Pediatr Psychol 2011;36(9): 1017–29.

77. Grigg-Damberger M, Ralls F. Treatment strategies for complex behavioral insomnia in children with neurodevelopmental disorders. Curr Opin Pulm Med 2013;19:616–25.

78. Moon EC, Corkum P, Smith IM. Case study: a case-series evaluation of a behavioral sleep intervention for three children with autism and primary insomnia. J Pediatr Psychol 2011;36(1):47–54.

79. Weiskop S, Richdale A, Matthews J. Behavioural treatment to reduce sleep problems in children with autism or fragile X syndrome. Dev Med Child Neurol 2005;47(2):94–104.

80. Wolf M, Risley T, Mees H. Application of operant conditioning procedures to the behavior problems of an autistic child. Behav Res Ther 1964; 1:305–12.

81. Durand VM, Gernet-Dott P, Mapstone E. Treatment of sleep disorders in children with developmental disabilities. J Assoc Pers Sev Handicaps 1996; 21(3):114–22.

82. Moore PS. The use of social stories in a psychology service for children with learning disabilities: a case study of a sleep problem. Bri J Learn Disabil 2004;32(3):133–8.

83. Howlin P. A brief report on the elimination of long term sleeping problems in a 6-yr-old autistic boy. Behav Psychother 1984;12(3):257–60.

84. Reed HE, McGrew SG, Artibee K, et al. Parent-based sleep education workshops in autism. J Child Neurol 2009;24(8):936–45.

85. DeLeon IG, Fisher WW, Marhefka J. Decreasing self-injurious behavior associated with awakening in a child with autism and developmental delays. Behav Interv 2004;19(2):111–9.

86. Piazza CC, Fisher WW, Sherer M. Treatment of multiple sleep problems in children with developmental disabilities: faded bedtime with response cost versus bedtime scheduling. Dev Med Child Neurol 1997;39(6):414–8.

87. Christodulu KV, Durand VM. Reducing bedtime disturbance and night waking using positive bedtime routines and sleep restriction. Focus Autism Other Dev Stud 2004;19(3):130–9.

88. Durand VM, Christodulu KV, Koegel RL. Description of a sleep-restriction program to reduce bedtime disturbances and night waking. J Posit Behav Interv 2004;6(2):83–91.

89. Sadeh A. Cognitive-behavioral treatment for childhood sleep disorders. Clin Psychol Rev 2005; 25(5):612–28.

90. Tikotzky L, Sadeh A. The role of cognitive–behavioral therapy in behavioral childhood insomnia. Sleep Med 2010;11(7):686–91.

91. Bessey M, Coulombe JA, Smith IM, et al. Assessing parental sleep attitudes and beliefs in typically developing children and children with ADHD and ASD. Child Health Care 2013;42(2):116–33.

92. Bell BG, Belsky J. Parents, parenting, and children's sleep problems: exploring reciprocal effects. Br J Dev Psychol 2008;26(4):579–93.

93. Malow BA, Adkins KW, Reynolds A, et al. Parent-based sleep education for children with autism spectrum disorders. J Autism Dev Disord 2014; 44(1):216–28.

94. Phillips L, Appleton RE. Systematic review of melatonin treatment in children with neurodevelopmental disabilities and sleep impairment. Dev Med Child Neurol 2004;46(11):771–5.

95. Rossignol DA, Frye RE. Melatonin in autism spectrum disorders: a systematic review and meta-analysis. Dev Med Child Neurol 2011;53:783.

96. Guénolé F, Godbout R, Nicolas A, et al. Melatonin for disordered sleep in individuals with autism spectrum disorders: systematic review and discussion. Sleep Med Rev 2011;15(6):379–87.

97. Bendz LM, Scates AC. Melatonin treatment for insomnia in pediatric patients with attention-deficit/hyperactivity disorder. Ann Pharmacother 2010;44:185–91.

98. Hoebert M, van der Heijden KB, van Geijlswijk IM, et al. Long-term follow-up of melatonin treatment in children with ADHD and chronic sleep onset insomnia. J Pineal Res 2009;47(1):1–7.

99. Ahmareen O, Neary E, Sharif F. Sleep disorders in children with developmental delay. Int J Disabil Hum Dev 2013. Available at: http://degruyter.com/view/j/ijdhd.ahead-of-print/ijdhd-2013-0025/ijdhd-2013-0025.xml. Accessed December 10, 2013.

100. Hollway JA, Aman MG. Pharmacological treatment of sleep disturbance in developmental disabilities: a review of the literature. Res Dev Disabil 2011; 32(3):939–62.

101. Johnson KP, Malow BA. Assessment and pharmacologic treatment of sleep disturbance in autism. Child Adolesc Psychiatr Clin N Am 2008;17(4): 773–85.

102. Barrett JR, Tracy DK, Giaroli G. To sleep or not to sleep: a systematic review of the literature of pharmacological treatments of insomnia in children and adolescents with attention-deficit/hyperactivity disorder. J Child Adolesc Psychopharmacol 2013; 23(10):1–8.

Application of Cognitive Behavioral Therapy for Insomnia in the Pediatric Population

Daniel S. Lewin, PhD, DABSM, CBSM*

KEYWORDS

- Child and adolescent • Insomnia • Cognitive behavioral therapy • Pathophysiology
- Sleep problems

KEY POINTS

- There is a significant gap in the literature defining child and adolescent insomnias and their pathophysiology.
- Developing clinically useful definitions is particularly important because there is evidence that a significant number of children have sleep problems. Definitions of the disorder and pathophysiology may also provide important insights into the origin of insomnia in adults.
- Four categories of child and adolescent insomnia are proposed: idiopathic insomnia, insomnia associated with hyperarousal and mild affective disturbance, acquired insomnia, and insomnia associated with persistent medical and mental health problems.
- Although there have been no published reports on the efficacy of cognitive behavior therapy for insomnia (CBTI) in children, many components are applicable to children and are described in detail.
- Future directions for research on child and adolescent insomnia include basic definitions of the disorder, pathophysiology, and the efficacy of CBTI and modifications adapted for this age group.

INTRODUCTION

The behavioral insomnias of childhood (BIC) are a distinct category of sleep disorders that have been extensively studied and are, for the most part, well defined. Over the past several decades, several well-validated and highly efficacious treatment protocols for the BIC that focus on young children (ages 6 months to 5 years) have also been developed,[1] and the use of cognitive behavior therapy for insomnia in adults (CBTI) has been well documented.[2] However, the definitions, pathophysiology, and treatment of insomnia in school-aged children and adolescents are still evolving and there is some controversy about how they should be defined and whether they differ fundamentally from adult insomnia.

Given that numerous studies have found a high prevalence of insomnia both in healthy children and in those with psychiatric comorbidities such as anxiety, depression, and autism spectrum disorders,[3,4] there is clearly a need both for a better understanding of the nature of and causal factors in childhood and adolescent insomnia (CHAI) and for evidence-based treatments. However, there have been few studies that have evaluated the efficacy of protocols or individual techniques for the treatment of insomnia in older children and adolescents.[5] This article focuses on proposed definitions of CHAI and theories about its origin and

Conflict of Interest: None.
Pediatric Sleep Medicine, Children's National Medical Center, 111 Michigan Avenue, North West, Washington, DC 20010, USA
* Sleep and Pulmonary Medicine, Children's National Medical Center, Washington, DC 20010.
E-mail address: dlewin@childrensnational.org

Sleep Med Clin 9 (2014) 169–180
http://dx.doi.org/10.1016/j.jsmc.2014.03.003

pathophysiology. These are followed by a review of the components of the CBTI intervention and their usefulness in treatment of CHAI. Methods of delivery and cases are used as examples of the approaches to intervention. In addition, future directions for intervention modalities and research are discussed.

DEFINITIONS OF CHAI

In both the Diagnostic and Statistical Manual of Mental Disorders, Fifth Edition,[6] and the International Classification of Sleep Disorders, Third edition (ICSD-3), the traditional definition of insomnia remains essentially unchanged (ie, persistent difficulty with sleep initiation, duration, consolidation, or quality that occurs despite adequate opportunity and circumstances for sleep, and resulting in some form of daytime impairment). However, in the ICSD-3, compared with previous versions, the designation of primary versus secondary insomnias is no longer included and the complex and specific insomnia subtype classification scheme has been abandoned. There are now 3 basic diagnostic categories for insomnia largely based on duration of symptoms: chronic insomnia disorder, short-term insomnia disorder, and other insomnia disorder. These diagnoses apply to patients with and without comorbidities. Although BIC and its subtypes (limit setting sleep disorder and sleep onset association disorder) have been subsumed under the general category of insomnia, the definition of insomnia has now been expanded to include parent/caregiver report of sleep disturbances and associated impairments in daytime function in the child and caregiver(s).

As an alternative conceptualization of diagnostic categories of CHAI, and recognizing their diverse causes and pathophysiology, some general subtypes may be proposed, such as idiopathic, affective, learned, and comorbid with a medical/psychiatric/neurodevelopmental condition or trauma. The first category may be viewed as the one that is closest to previous definitions of idiopathic insomnia, namely difficulties with sleep onset, maintenance, and quality that have their origin in childhood and are not clearly linked to some precipitating cause. Although all insomnias involve psychophysiologic activation or hyperarousal both during the sleep period and across the day, idiopathic insomnia may be construed as more trait based rather than learned hyperarousal. The idiopathic subtype should be differentiated from insomnias that have their origin in affective disturbance. The affective subtype includes nighttime anxiety and mild daytime anxiety and includes worries and rumination about sleep,

performance in school, social interactions, and so forth, which do not meet criteria for an affective disorder. These patients may also have a history of more significant mood disturbance that has resolved. The third subtype is learned or acquired insomnia. Here the initial presentation may be that of behavioral insomnia of childhood, a circadian rhythm disorder that emerges during adolescence, or a life event that leads to acute changes in sleep habits that then persist over time. These changes may in turn result in the patient and/or parents adopting compensatory sleep-related strategies that are ultimately counterproductive (eg, lying in bed awake for long periods, daytime napping) and result in a deterioration of sleep quality. The fourth subtype is characterized by persistent insomnia symptoms that are secondary to medical, psychiatric, and developmental disorders (eg, autism spectrum disorders) and/or iatrogenic (eg, psychotropic medication) effects.

The discussion of CBTI in children and adolescents in this article is based on this conceptual nosology of CHAI subtypes: idiopathic insomnia, learned/acquired insomnia, insomnia associated with mild affective disturbance, and comorbid insomnia with the recognition that there is often overlap among these categories. Based on clinical experience, a CBTI treatment package or selected elements may be efficacious for all these subtypes of insomnia. However, the presence of additional symptoms and causal factors may require the use of more focused assessments, selected intervention targets based on associated treatment outcome variables, and adjunctive treatment modalities.

ASSESSMENT OF CHAI

The specific targets of treatment of CHAI include (1) presleep habits that interfere with wake-to-sleep transitions and sleep onset; (2) dysfunctional beliefs and cognitions associated with sleep; (3) psychophysiologic arousal associated with bedtime; and (4) other behaviors negatively affecting sleep continuity and daytime functions such as caregiver-child interactions during the sleep period, multiple arousals during sleep, early morning awakenings, daytime sleep, and irregular sleep-wake schedules. A thorough clinical interview should target all of these domains.

Standardized questionnaires for child and adolescent sleep problems can assist in diagnosis and identification of specific problem areas. However, there are gaps in age groups covered by these questionnaires, particularly in children more than 12 years of age. The most widely used questionnaires in pediatric clinic settings are the Children's Sleep Habits Questionnaire[7] and the

Sleep Habits Survey for Adolescents.[8] The most widely used adult questionnaire, the Pittsburgh Sleep Quality Index, has not been validated in the pediatric population, but may be useful in older adolescents. The recently developed patient reported outcome measure information system (PROMIS) measures, which have been developed for children and adolescents primarily for research, may also be good tools because they provide continuity for all age groups and also include measures of psychopathology.[9,10]

Sleep logs or diaries are also critically important tools in the assessment of insomnia. As completed by either caregivers or older children and adolescents, they provide a subjective overview of sleep-wake patterns for 1 to 2 weeks and provide some of the richest clinical data on sleep-wake habits and, in some cases, reasonable estimates of sleep-wake periods. Key variables that may be derived from sleep logs include sleep period variability and midsleep time (an estimate of circadian phase), total sleep time, wake time after sleep onset, sleep efficiency (ratio of time asleep to time in bed), and daytime napping.

COMPONENTS OF CBTI IN CHAI
Bedtime Routines and Rituals

Bedtime routines and rituals provide predictable cues and familiarity and help to establish the optimal milieu for the letting down of vigilance and relaxation, which are both prerequisites for a smooth transition from wake to sleep. Routines and rituals are particularly important because the period before bedtime is further complicated by a burst in vigilance known as the forbidden zone,[11] which may have served to help early humans prepare a safe sleep environment during a period when they were susceptible to the attacks of nocturnal predators. At different stages of development and for different children these cues serve various purposes. Most preschool and school-aged children benefit from having a predictable and controlled environment. Not knowing what to expect can increase activation and arousal, and in some cases anxiety, in both young children and older children. Such activation can delay sleep and cause stressful interactions between parents and children. For example, when children do not know what to expect, they test the limits of what is acceptable. When the caregiver responds with clear and supportive limit setting that requires the child to self-regulate, the testing of limits gradually dissipates over a few minutes or a few days. However, when the caregiver's response is unclear, or laced with emotion (frustration, anger) or ambivalence, children's negative behavior is reinforced and they continue to test limits. This process

describes the classic pattern of parent-child interactions that is central to the BIC in young children, but may persist in older children and be an important contributor to the emergence and persistence of CHAI.

Although hypothetical, the origins of insomnia in childhood may be categorized as either poor regulation of emotion and behavior (ie, affective disturbance subtype) or chronic reinforcement of the child's acting out, limit testing, and attention-seeking behavior at bedtime. When any of these problems occur, the child may be labeled by the family as a poor sleeper (ie, learned insomnia). In the long term, poor affect regulation and being labeled a poor sleeper may result in persistent problems with wake-to-sleep transitions.

Although school-aged children may have a history of sleep problems, they may also develop de novo sleep problems that meet criteria for CHAI. There are many underlying initiating causes that are important to understand because they may help to guide treatment planning. As school-aged children develop more knowledge and experience with cause-and-effect relationships, they can apply their developing cognitive skills to the regulation of their state of arousal. They have the skills to set and test out their own limits and have internalized their caregivers responses whether optimal (ie, consistent, rationale, loving, supportive) or not. With the development of cognitive skills, as well as exposure to environmental influences such as media and more complex narratives, comes imagination. Imagination and complex narratives are often woven together into frightening or overly stimulating threads that can increase cognitive activation and interfere with sleep onset. This presleep arousal associated with actual or perceived fears can become habitual. High sleep drive and tiredness can contribute to disinhibition and, if coupled with a natural period of hypervigilance (also called the forbidden zone[12]), can lead to long periods of wakefulness at sleep onset and in the middle of the night.

Adolescents may have carried forward any of these problems and habits, but have a couple of additional challenges. The first is a hunger for novelty and stimulation that is often social, sometimes sexual, and frequently involves thrill seeking. These sensation-seeking and accompanying risk-taking behaviors are not only further exacerbated by chronic sleep loss but often are coupled with high academic and other demands and changes in circadian regulation; circumstances that create fertile ground for poor sleep habits. Moreover, increased use on electronics during adolescence, which serve as a highly effective and efficient conduit for virtual and real-time access, in turn to highly stimulating material reinforces delayed sleep onset.

Rituals and routines that are age appropriate are important in establishing a safe and predicable environment. Limiting personal narratives that can quickly spin into fear-laced, dysfunctional, or activating cognitive threads and decreasing exciting and thrill seeking and even addictive behavior (eg, gaming, social media) are equally important. However, delineating age-appropriate routines can be challenging because interests, sensitivities, and family values complicate the matter. For example, for some families, a bedroom featuring every conceivable category of electronics is a status symbol, whereas for others the lack of access to a television in the home is a point of pride. For other families, praying together for deceased relatives is a bedtime ritual even if it is distressing for a young child; for still others, the bedroom is viewed as the adolescent's sanctuary and parents never set foot in it in order to monitor their child's behavior. Positive rituals and routines can cue feelings of security and safety and serve to distract and quiet an active and imaginative mind.

Education

Education is a key component of CBTI and most sleep interventions, are intended to correct misconceptions, decrease worry, and provide a reality check for dysfunctional expectations.[13] Understanding normal sleep patterns and having reasonable expectations with regard to developmentally appropriate sleep behaviors are helpful for both parents and children. Key components of education include sleep needs and timing a circadian regulation across development, the function of sleep, definitions of sleep disorders and problems, the rationale for specific interventions and what to expect as treatment progresses.[14,15] Education addresses misconceptions and cognitive distortions that can be a focus of obsessive worry. For example, the importance of sleep continuity should be addressed early in treatment; specifically, the normal sleep period is not necessarily continuous and may include multiple brief awakenings (eg, a few seconds to a few minutes) and at least one longer awakening.[16–18] These awakenings often occur at transitions from one sleep stage to another. More extended awakenings can occur after the homeostatic sleep drive for delta (non–rapid eye movement stage 3) sleep is satisfied during the first 4 to 6 hours of the sleep period.[19–21] The concept of first and second sleep helps to explain short and extended nighttime awakening and changes in the quality and perception of sleep across the night as well as the increased difficulty of returning to sleep after an early morning awakening.[22,23]

Education about optimal sleep timing and duration are also key to understanding the relationship between the inability to fall asleep or to obtain good-quality sleep and the schedule and sleep period. The simplest approach to amplifying the nighttime sleep drive is to eliminate daytime naps. Consideration of normal developmental changes is key: sleep parameters such as bedtimes, wake times, and sleep duration vary across childhood and adolescence and the failure to appreciate and incorporate these biologically based variations may contribute to symptoms of insomnia.

Educating patients and families about the rationale for specific interventions can also improve adherence to treatment protocols, motivate patients, provide them with more control over the course of treatment, and assist them in maintaining treatment gains. Providing patients with reasonable expectations about the course of treatment establishes realistic expectations and reduces disappointment and frustration when typical setbacks occur. It is common for patients and caregivers to enter treatment with the certainty that they have read everything and tried everything. When queried, however, many of the interventions have only been attempted for a short periods of time before being prematurely abandoned; this is often because of the so-called extinction response burst (ie, a regression to baseline behaviors) that frequently follows the initiation of a behavioral intervention. Teaching patients to expect an extinction response burst is also key because a setback after a few days of gains can undermine faith in a treatment plan.[1] Patients benefit from the understanding that persistence and maintaining gains for a week or more is necessary.

Healthy Sleep Practices Training

Training in healthy sleep practices (also called sleep hygiene) is a form of education in which the focus is on specific behaviors and habits that either support or interfere with sleep.[24,25] Many positive sleep practices use common sense that most people use on their own; others require discipline and effort to incorporate them in the daily routine and make them habitual. Healthy sleep practices in children and families are the same as those recommended for adults.[24,26] Key components include eliminating caffeine (iced tea, sodas, energy drinks, chocolate); engaging in quiet activities and using no electronic media within an hour of bedtime; removing or covering clocks in the bedroom; making the bedroom a comfortable and safe environment; eliminating noise, shadows, and other objects that may spark imagination, but allowing appropriate night lights, white noise, or relaxation sound recordings; using the bed only for sleep; and establishing a regular sleep/wake schedule that is age appropriate.

The optimal sleep schedule is based on age, individual preference, and environmental factors, such as parental work schedules, school start times, and extracurricular activities. Considering and prioritizing sleep and these other factors is a complex process and, in many homes, there is not an optimal plan but rather a best option. The tools to arrive at the best plan include a 2-week sleep log or diary and a thorough interview of the child and family to determine priorities and the diversity of demands. The highest priority consideration should be the child's level of function, including daytime tiredness and sleep propensity (ie, frequency and duration of planned and unplanned daytime sleep), and impairments of mood, attention, and social relationships. Key sleep log variables include sleep onset latency, time into bed, total sleep time, wake time after sleep onset, sleep efficiency, wake time and midsleep time (ie, the midpoint of the sleep period, which is a unitary marker of sleep period variability and an estimate of chronotype).[27] Chronotype becomes increasingly important as the child ages because there is a trend for a phase delay at the time of puberty[28]; some consideration of the individual's ability to adapt to variability in sleep timing and duration is also an imperative.[29]

Perhaps the most challenging issue to navigate with children and their families is prioritizing sleep among all the other child-specific and family demands; motivation to sleep on an optimal schedule and to implement optimal sleep practices is often overridden by other factors. In these situations, the clinician's skills in motivational interviewing and helping parents to set limits on problematic behaviors (eg, use of electronic devices, gaming, and social media) are critical. Borrowing principles of other behavior change programs, an incremental approach can be successful. For example, giving up social media activities at bedtime, which may be the primary social time teens have during the week, can be daunting, but agreeing to give it up for a weekend or a week is more palatable. Encouraging children to engage their social networks by challenging friends to follow the same rules and sleep schedule for a short period of time can be strategic and may result in some maintenance of gains. In addition, it is important to stress to the patient that the outcome of these changes (ie, improved sleep quality and better control of the sleep-wake cycle) can be intrinsically rewarding.

Some poor sleep hygiene practices, such as use of social and electronic media, may become deeply entrenched habits or may arise from individuals' attempts to compensate for their inability to initiate or maintain sleep. During the past several decades there has been a significant increase in the use of electronic media use by children at bedtime and after lights-out.[30] Based on clinical practice observations, it is common for children to wake in the middle of their sleep periods and use electronic media, or awaken too early in the morning because they want extra screen time. Because such practices represent potent sleep disruptors, children (and parents) should not have access to electronic media in the bedroom and should not use devices within 30 minutes of the sleep period in both the evening and morning.

Clocks in the bedroom may also function as a significant sleep disruptor, because they can cue frustration and increase psychophysiologic activation. Patients with insomnia often check bedroom clocks repeatedly both at the beginning and in the middle of the night to assess the passage of time awake. Giving up this behavior can facilitate the letting down of vigilance and arousal and thus facilitate smoother sleep transitions.

The timing of eating and exercise are also a focus of healthy sleep practices. Optimal nutrition and exercise may improve sleep quality; but having large meals, going to bed hungry, or engaging in aerobic exercise in close proximity to bedtime are all potential sleep disruptors. Other sleep recommendations focus on eliminating behaviors and activities at or around bedtime or in bed that are activating or that increase stress and worry, such as reading material that is overly stimulating, doing homework, or engaging in other tasks that increase worry or frustration. Optimal bedtime or middle-of-the-night activities should involve with a moderate demand on attention and focus that serve to distract from negative and activating cognitions (eg, listening to quiet music, doing puzzles).

Cognitive Interventions

Disruptive cognitions that are common in children with insomnia may be divided into a few different categories. Bedtime fears are particularly prominent and may persist through adolescence with content ranging from monsters to real or perceived fears of home break-ins, and harm or illness of family members. Fears that are in the realm of imagination and perceived threats occur more frequently in children who have a tendency to be hypervigilant or anxious. These fears may start with mild discomfort associated with being alone in bed or with the natural circadian-mediated increase in vigilance (the forbidden zone) that occurs before sleep onset. Habitual worry at bedtime may lead to an escalation in fears, which caregivers may then reinforce by coming into the child's bedroom or otherwise providing excessive attention. Heightened arousal associated with actual threats (eg, living in a dangerous neighborhood or a history of trauma or abuse) are particularly challenging to address and may need additional cognitive and relaxation techniques and parental/patient reassurance. Whether real, perceived, or imagined, fears link mental and physiologic arousal. Furthermore, both fears and worry during the bedtime and sleep period are thought to be unmasked or amplified by the dulling of executive function that is caused by inadequate sleep. In addition, worry at bedtime may be specifically linked to the sleep period or occur throughout the day and at bedtime; the latter more strongly suggests a global anxiety disorder (eg, social or generalized anxiety) or a depressive disorder.

The second category of cognitive problems is those that are primarily focused on the consequences of inadequate sleep, tiredness, and fatigue. Periodic or excessive worry about nighttime sleep during the day may lead to increased cognitive arousal at night and become a self-fulfilling prophecy. Within a family unit, repeated labeling of one individual as a poor sleeper can further reinforce the predictive power by assigning a role to the identified individual and worsen cognitive arousal at bedtime. All of these factors may maintain the problematic behaviors and cognitions.

Cognitive therapy interventions are intended to decrease mental arousal, correct misconceptions, eliminate habitual fears and worry, and uncouple cognitive and physiologic arousal.[31,32] The first step in any intervention is to identify the target cognitions and determine the attitude of patients and their families toward changing them.[33] The next step is to challenge and correct misconceptions, such as pathologizing normal brief night wakings and using napping to offset reduced nighttime sleep. The third step is patient and/or caregiver-assisted monitoring of the frequency of the dysfunctional cognitions using a checklist or diary. Worry time, which provides an opportunity for circumscribed and limited worrying, should not occur just before bedtime because this may increase cognitive arousal.

The following is an example of a dialogue from a therapy session that demonstrates a straightforward approach to identification, discussion, and challenge of fears and misconceptions associated with insomnia.

Case example 1

This 10-year-old girl presents to a sleep clinic with difficulty initiating sleep every night of the week (sleep onset latency ranging from 30–120 minutes), multiple callouts to parents, and frequent check-ins with parents in their bedroom, both at the beginning and middle of the night.

Patient: I am scared that someone is going to break into my house and kidnap my sister and me.

Clinician: Do you have any other nighttime fears?

Patient: Sometimes I worry that my parents are going to leave us alone in the house and I have to check on them and see where they are and what they are doing.

Clinician: Is it possible that your parents would leave you and your sister alone in the house?

Patient: No! But I'm still scared and I have to know where they are.

Clinician: Can you think of a reason why your parents might urgently need to leave the house at night?

Patient: Well maybe to walk the dog? But that would be OK I guess, because they leave us alone when they visit with our next door neighbors or walk the dog during the day.

Clinician: How safe is your neighborhood? Has anything bad ever happened? For example, a break-in?

Patient: ...No, well, I saw on the news that someone was breaking into houses in another neighborhood.

Clinician: How common do you think it is that there are break-ins near where you live?

Patient: (looks at parents for their input). I don't know, but I worry about it.

Father: Honey, there has never been a break-in in our neighborhood and we set the alarm every night. Plus, what would be the first thing that would happen if someone were to try to break in?

Patient: Sunshine would bark.

Mother: ...and wake us up and we would make sure that everything is OK.

Clinician: Do you need to worry about break-ins or your parent leaving you and your sister alone?

Patient: No...but I do.

Mother: ...I didn't know that she has these fears, but she does come out of the bedroom and call us to her bedroom repeatedly to ask if the alarm is on, and then often asks other questions that seem pretty random...

This dialogue demonstrates how, in just a brief period, fears may be identified, challenged, and deflated. Parents' involvement in the dialogue, observation of the clinician's approach to querying, and hearing their child articulate her fears goes a long way toward decreasing the potency of the fears and improving parents' skills in responding to the fears. The fears and misconceptions are addressed by convincing the child that the threats are exceedingly low probability events, are not ultimately under her control, and are therefore not worthy of focused time and energy. Some fears and cognitions are more tenacious and may require more challenges overtime in therapy and tracking and monitoring as homework.

Relaxation and Mindfulness-based Techniques

This diverse set of techniques is effective in reducing vigilance and decreasing or reducing the impact of fear, worry, and other maladaptive cognitions,[34–36] including those that intrude on the bedtime and sleep period.[37–42] These interventions have been shown to be effective in pediatric populations in guided exposure therapies for anxiety and in managing chronic or procedural pain.[43–45] All of these techniques have the common goal of focusing attention on physical sensation or mental activity in the present moment; they also uncouple the link between mental and physiologic arousal.[46] Breathing techniques may have the added benefit of improving oxygen exchange, decreasing heart rate, and reducing blood pressure.

One advantage of these interventions is that the benefits are immediate; this is because experiencing even momentary relaxation or distraction is reinforcing. In contrast, the associated benefits may be temporary and are not immediately effective with cognitions that are habitual and have been in place for a long time. In addition, effective use of the techniques requires practice. Encouraging parents and children to practice together and monitoring the frequency of practice are important steps in developing skills and integrating these interventions into daily life.

In practice it may be optimal to introduce a child and family to a menu of techniques and ask them to rate the effectiveness of each. Because breathing exercises have immediate physiologic effects and are the starting point for many of the other interventions, they may be the best entry point. Another good initial intervention is sensate focusing (eg, observing the temperature of the breath, and parts of body that move when you breathe), which is easy to introduce

and is a primary component of other relaxation and mindfulness-based techniques. Other standard techniques include progressive muscle relaxation,[47,48] guided imagery, or other mental relaxation and focusing techniques.[49] The following is script for a basic introduction to these techniques.

Case example 2
Script for Relaxation Intervention

Everyone find a comfortable seat, close your eyes, and place your hands palm up or palm down on your thighs. Begin by observing your breathing. Do not do anything, but just become aware of the movement of your chest and tummy. You may also observe that other parts of your body move when you breathe: your shoulders, back, and neck. Now focus on the air as it passes through your nose. Think about the temperature of the air as it moves in your nose and out. Where in your nose do you feel the change in temperature? Focus on the humidity of the air, dry and cool when you inhale and warm and moist when you exhale. Now we will change our focus to the breath and make some very slight changes in how we breathe. As you breathe in, count slowly from 1 to 4 and hold the breath for 1 count; then breathe out on a slow count of 6 and pause for 1 count once you have exhaled all the air. Let's practice. [Clinician should repeat practice, watching participants, until certain that all have the technique]. Repeat this on your own, counting to yourself.

Now we are going to focus on sound. Try to listen just to the sounds inside this room. Ignore the sounds outside the room. You can do this by listening very carefully to the sounds and the different qualities of each sound. Can you hear others breathing, the sound of the air handler, the computer fan? Can you hear different pitches, pulsations, other qualities?

Now allow yourself to forget the sounds in the room and focus only on sounds outside the room. If you hear voices, try to imagine who is speaking and what they are talking about. If you hear a car, try to imagine the type of car and who might be driving it. You will notice that your attention will automatically shift to sounds that you are trying to ignore or even to other thoughts about your day or what you are going to do next. These shifts get fewer as you practice, but it is important to understand that these shifts are the same as the intrusive thoughts that occur when you lie in bed and try to fall asleep.

(*continued on next page*)

**Case example 2
(continued)**

Now, again focus on your breath and body. Notice whether your attention has been focused or has jumped around. Notice whether your attention is on something you worry about, for example, whether you have to be next to a friend in school or first in line, or some other concern.

As you learn the skills of focusing you will be able to focus for longer and longer periods of time and you will experience fewer distractions. Do not let distractions or worries frustrate you; that is how the brain works. Instead notice that it is comforting and relaxing to be able to focus on something other than your usual daily worries. Think about how you focused on the sounds inside and outside the room. Recall each time your attention shifted away and then shifted back. Eventually, you will be able to focus away from your thoughts and worries that occur at bedtime.

You told me previously that you play [instrument or sport]. We will now do an exercise that is good for relaxation and also can improve your skills in your favorite activities. Imagine yourself holding your [eg, baseball bat or violin], feel the weight and texture of the object, see whether you can see some of the smallest details such as the wood grain, the texture, some lettering. Now imagine yourself assuming the perfect position, poised to play. Now imagine moving through your activity in the slowest of slow motion.

This series of techniques can be introduced in any order. The goal is to identify techniques that engage children's intrinsic interests and help them to be observers of their internal states and to focus their attention. By learning to notice when their focus shifts away from what is intended and toward typical distractions (daytime worries, fears, self-criticism), patients can apply the same techniques when lying in bed unable to sleep.

Behavioral Interventions

Behavioral approaches to treatment of insomnia are both complimentary to cognitive techniques and necessary components of treatment. Although the cognitive techniques shift focus from activating cognitions that increase vigilance, the behavioral techniques eliminate learned associations and environmental reinforcement. The components that are relevant to children are stimulus control, modification of patterns of parental reinforcement, sleep restriction, and bedtime fading.

Stimulus control is a classic behavioral intervention that first identifies and then dissociates a stimulus from an established response that interferes with healthy function.[50] In the treatment of insomnia, the classic stimulus response associations are the bed and the psychophysiologic activation that includes worry, fears, increased vigilance, and physiologic manifestations such as increased heart and respiratory rate, muscle tension, and other more general somaticized tension. The typical instruction is for an individual to limit awake-time in bed. Between 15 and 20 minutes of wakefulness in bed is the maximum recommended time. Patients should be taught to identify increased vigilance, frustration, and/or general psychophysiologic activation as the cues to get out of bed and sit quietly in the bedroom or somewhere else in the home. When practiced regularly, this intervention disassociates the cues between the bed or bedroom and psychophysiologic activation.

Caregiver reinforcement of children's problematic behaviors, and particularly of their attempts to repeatedly engage the parent at bedtime, is one of the most potent initiating and sustaining causes of childhood insomnia and is an important target of intervention. These reinforced patterns of behavior interfere with the child's wake-to-sleep transitions and place a high demand on caregivers' time. Although patterns of social behavior are not a focus of most standard CBTI interventions with adults, they are a critical addition to interventions for pediatric patients and a brief review is provided here.

The principles used to modify reinforcement are the same as those in standard interventions for BIC; these are well validated in children less than 6 years of age.[1] As is the case with most interventions discussed here, there is no research on the efficacy of these interventions in children older than 6 years. However, many of the same interventions for younger children may be applied in older children, although modifications are needed for adolescents. The first step is the identification of parent/child interactions that delay bedtime, increase psychophysiologic arousal, or involve conflict (eg, repeated caregiver reminders that the child should calm down, prepare for bed, stay in the bedroom, and not call out). Because the child's interactions with the parent often involve fears, worries, and faulty assumptions or myths about sleep and sleep capacity, cognitive interventions should be used concurrently with behavioral interventions.

The first step in the implementation of the behavioral treatment approach is having the parent and child identify the problematic behavior patterns and then monitor them. Immediate, gradual, or graduated elimination of parental interactions reduce the frequency of the child's attempts to engage the parent. Flexibility is required to coordinate (1) reinforcement of the more positive caregiver-child interactions associated with the sleep period with (2) approaches to decreasing cognitive arousal through cognitive and relaxation therapy. There is great variability in individuals' and families' abilities to implement these different techniques and acquire skill in using them. There is often emergence of persistent fears or tenacious attachment to familiar and dysfunctional behavior patterns. Sometimes these are related to maintaining routines within a family; for example, how caregivers parcel out attention to siblings. Sometimes minor changes in interactions between parents and one child can have a far-reaching impact on family dynamics. Either anticipating these changes or attending to them during the course of therapy is important for the implementation and maintenance of treatment gains.

Sleep restriction is a core component of CBTI for adults[51,52] and although it has not been studied as an intervention for CHAI, the principles are relevant to this age group and it is commonly used in clinical practice. Sleep restriction involves determining the patient's average sleep time over the course of 1, but optimally 2, prior weeks. A simple average of sleep time, based on a 2-week sleep log, should be the basis for establishing a nightly sleep duration. Although the recommended sleep period is typically shorter than what is optimal based on development stage and perceived need, sleep restriction serves to increase the sleep drive and facilitates implementation of stimulus control. Once sleep efficiency improves, sleep duration can be gradually increased by intervals of 10 to 15 minutes. Following sleep hygiene recommendations and eliminating all but one daytime nap that is less than 20 minutes are also critical in increasing the nighttime sleep drive.

Bedtime fading is a different type of intervention but is also an important compliment to both sleep restriction and stimulus control. Again, based on reports on a sleep log, patients are instructed to shift their bedtime to the average time that they typically fall asleep, which matches bedtime with the time that the child is currently physiologically ready for sleep. Once sleep efficiency improves, then the bedtime can gradually be advanced.

Case example 3

JB is a 9-year-old boy who has a history of difficulty initiating and maintaining sleep, but is otherwise healthy and doing well in third grade. He tends to be obsessive about getting his homework done and he rechecks his work until his parents reassure him that he has done a good job. He has a close friend, but frequently complains that other children say mean things about him. He is a top scorer on his soccer team. He has 7-year-old brother who is extremely social and easy going. JB has always had trouble falling asleep. He becomes extremely fearful at night and sometimes becomes extremely agitated and panics if he is not allowed to sleep with another family member. He starts talking about sleeping arrangements in the afternoon and sometimes negotiates with his younger brother or does extra chores in exchange for bedroom sharing arrangements. When queried, he mentioned no specific fears aside from some minor worries about school performance, interactions with his peers and occasionally about his home being broken into or some other catastrophic event. On his own initiative, he stopped watching television because he is scared of seeing frightening advertisements and shows.

The treatment approach for JB involved identifying daytime fears about sleep and monitoring their frequency and intensity. He agreed that his fears were irrational. He was able to identify feelings of panic that started around his sternum and spread up to his throat when thinking about sleep and while lying alone in bed at night. His parents were instructed to spend 10 minutes with him in the afternoon completing a log of sleep-related thoughts and fears and a worry diary. He was taught deep breathing, sensate focusing, and guided imagery that involve taking soccer penalty shots in slow motion. His parents acknowledged that they had reinforced his fears by spending a great deal of time talking about his sleep and getting involved in mediating negotiations about sleeping arrangements. They all agreed to 1 approach to sleeping arrangements that would no longer be a topic of discussion or negotiation. He committed to staying in his own bedroom for at least 2 weeks. His parents agreed to check in on him at the beginning of the night on a random reinforcement schedule based on what was convenient for them. If he woke in the middle of the night and could not fall asleep, he would be allowed to sleep on the floor in his parents' or brother's room as long as he did not wake them. In addition, JB agreed that he would not get into bed until he was tired and ready to fall asleep.

Case example 4

AS is a 14-year-old girl who is an accomplished musician and plays in the school and local community orchestras. Her grades in middle and high school have recently changed from As to Bs. She has a high drive to engage socially and has a small group of close friends. She has no history of significant medical problems aside from occasional gastrointestinal disturbance and headaches. AS and her parents agree that she has been a poor sleeper her whole life. Although she functions well in most domains, she is often tired during the day and longs to take a nap. She has tried putting her head down and closing her eyes in school and after school, but cannot fall asleep. She goes to bed between 9:30 and 10:00 PM and lies awake until 11:15 or 11:30 PM. She typically awakens twice each night and on a bad night can be awake for 2 hours. If she is still awake after 4:00 AM, she does not go back to sleep, but gets out of bed at 5:30 AM to prepare for school and get to the bus stop at 6:45 AM. When going to sleep at night, AS has a regular bedtime routine that ends with 20 minutes of social media while lying in bed. She turns out the lights and goes to sleep. On weekends she goes to bed by 1:00 AM and typically falls asleep within 10 to 15 minutes and then her parents allow her to sleep in, but never beyond 11:00 AM.

The treatment approach for AS involved schedule modification, stimulus control, sleep hygiene modifications, and changing the family mythology about her being a poor sleeper. Her sleep log was particularly instructive with a mean midsleep time of 2:30 AM on weeknights and 6:00 AM on weekends. She had a typical phase delay propensity and had developed many maladaptive strategies. It was also suspected that some of her early morning awakenings were brief and she had paradoxic insomnia (also known as sleep state misperception). She acknowledged that it was possible that she was actually asleep but perceived herself to be awake. After a review of key information about normal sleep-wake regulation, the primary interventions were sleep restriction to 7 hours, bedtime fading with an initial bedtime of 11:30 PM, and stimulus control. On weekends she was instructed to wake no later than 8:00 AM for at least 2 weeks, and to attempt to sleep in as late as possible on weekday mornings, which required her to lay out clothes, pack her backpack, and make her lunch the night before. She agreed to stop attempts at napping. She committed to learning relaxation techniques on her own and she and her parents agreed to monitor the family's cognitions regarding sleep. She was also instructed to keep a sleep log to record her progress.

SUMMARY

The diagnosis of insomnia in children and adolescents is controversial, and there are no studies that have evaluated CBTI in individuals 6 to 18 years of age. There is no reason to assume that the prevalence of CHAI, especially in adolescents, is significantly different from that in adults. With increasing demands on the time of children and their families, and the profusion of electronic media, it is likely that prevalence rates of CHAI may increase. However, the pathophysiology of CHAI has yet to be fully defined and it is likely that subtypes should be considered both as a means of prevention and the targeting of treatments. The application of all or at least some components of CBTI for CHAI with minor modifications (most often these involve the caregivers taking an active role) are probably already being practiced widely by pediatric, behavioral health, and sleep specialists in clinical settings. There is a need for valid definitions of sleep complaints among children as well as studies that evaluate the efficacy of CBTI for this age group.

REFERENCES

1. Mindell JA, Kuhn B, Lewin DS, et al, American Academy of Sleep Medicine. Behavioral treatment of bedtime problems and night wakings in infants and young children. Sleep 2006;29:1263–76 [Erratum appears in Sleep 2006;29(11):1380].
2. Chesson AL Jr, Anderson WM, Littner M, et al. Practice parameters for the nonpharmacologic treatment of chronic insomnia. An American Academy of Sleep Medicine report. Standards of Practice Committee of the American Academy of Sleep Medicine. Sleep 1999;22:1128–33.
3. Roberts RE, Roberts CR, Chan W. Ethnic differences in symptoms of insomnia among adolescents. Sleep 2006;29:359–65.
4. Roberts RE, Roberts CR, Chen IG. Impact of insomnia on future functioning of adolescents. J Psychosom Res 2002;53:561–9.
5. Tikotzky L, Sadeh A. The role of cognitive-behavioral therapy in behavioral childhood insomnia. Sleep Med 2010;11:686–91.
6. American Psychiatric Assocation. Diagnostic and statistical manual of mental disorders. 5th edition. Arlington, VA: American Psychiatric Assocation; 2013.

7. Owens JA, Spirito A, McGuinn M. The Children's Sleep Habits Questionnaire (CSHQ): psychometric properties of a survey instrument for school-aged children. Sleep 2000;23:1043–51.

8. Wolfson AR, Carskadon MA, Acebo C, et al. Evidence for the validity of a sleep habits survey for adolescents. Sleep 2003;26:213–6.

9. Arnedt JT. PROMIS of improved tools for assessing sleep and wake function: commentary on "Development of short forms from the PROMIS sleep disturbance and sleep-related impairment item banks". Behav Sleep Med 2011;10:25–7.

10. Yu L, Buysse DJ, Germain A, et al. Development of short forms from the PROMIS sleep disturbance and sleep-related impairment item banks. Behavioral Sleep Medicine 2011;10:6–24.

11. Ferber R. Solve your child's sleep problems. New York: Simon & Schuster; 1985.

12. Ferber R. Childhood sleep disorders. Neurol Clin 1996;14:493–511.

13. Morin CM, Culbert JP, Schwartz SM. Nonpharmacological interventions for insomnia: a meta-analysis of treatment efficacy. Am J Psychiatry 1994;151:1172–80.

14. Edinger JD, Wohlgemuth WK, Radtke RA, et al. Does cognitive-behavioral insomnia therapy alter dysfunctional beliefs about sleep? Sleep 2001;24:591–9.

15. Edinger JD, Sampson WS. A primary care "friendly" cognitive behavioral insomnia therapy. Sleep 2003;26:177–82.

16. Wehr TA. In short photoperiods, human sleep is biphasic. J Sleep Res 1992;1:103–7.

17. Owens JA, Spirito A, McGuinn M, et al. Sleep habits and sleep disturbance in elementary school-aged children. J Dev Behav Pediatr 2000;21:27–36.

18. Marcus CL, Omlin KJ, Basinki DJ, et al. Normal polysomnographic values for children and adolescents [see comment]. Am Rev Respir Dis 1992;146:1235–9.

19. Acebo C, Sadeh A, Seifer R, et al. Sleep/wake patterns derived from activity monitoring and maternal report for healthy 1- to 5-year-old children. Sleep 2005;28:1568–77.

20. Montgomery-Downs HE, O'Brien LM, Gulliver TE, et al. Polysomnographic characteristics in normal preschool and early school-aged children. Pediatrics 2006;117:741–53.

21. Porkka-Heiskanen T. Sleep homeostasis. Curr Opin Neurobiol 2013;23:799–805.

22. Ekrich R. At day's close. New York: WW Norton & Company; 2005. p. 416.

23. Hegarty S. The myth of the eight-hour sleep. In BBC news magazine. London (UK): BBC World Service; 2012.

24. Hauri P. The sleep disorder. M Kalamazoo, MI: Upjohn; 1982. p. 85.

25. Lacks P, Rotert M. Knowledge and practice of sleep hygiene techniques in insomniacs and good sleepers. Behav Res Ther 1986;24:365–8.

26. Billows M, Gradisar M, Dohnt H, et al. Family disorganization, sleep hygiene, and adolescent sleep disturbance. J Clin Child Adolesc Psychol 2009;38:745–52.

27. Lewy AJ. Melatonin and human chronobiology. Cold Spring Harb Symp Quant Biol 2007;72:623–36.

28. Carskadon MA, Vieira C, Acebo C. Association between puberty and delayed phase preference. Sleep 1993;16:258–62.

29. Spaeth AM, Goel N, Dinges DF. Managing neurobehavioral capability when social expediency trumps biological imperatives. Prog Brain Res 2012;199:377–98.

30. Cain N, Gradisar M. Electronic media use and sleep in school-aged children and adolescents: a review. Sleep Med 2010;11:735–42.

31. Morin CM, Bootzin RR, Buysse DJ, et al. Psychological and behavioral treatment of insomnia: update of the recent evidence (1998-2004). Sleep 2006;29:1398–414.

32. Morin CM. Insomnia: psychological assessment and management. New York: Guilford Press; 1993. p. 238.

33. Carney CE, Edinger JD, Morin CM, et al. Examining maladaptive beliefs about sleep across insomnia patient groups. J Psychosom Res 2010;68:57–65.

34. Goldin PR, Gross JJ. Effects of mindfulness-based stress reduction (MBSR) on emotion regulation in social anxiety disorder. Emotion 2010;10:83–91.

35. Jazaieri H, Goldin PR, Werner K, et al. A randomized trial of MBSR versus aerobic exercise for social anxiety disorder. J Clin Psychol 2012;68:715–31.

36. Seifert G, Kanitz JL, Pretzer K, et al. Improvement of circadian rhythm of heart rate variability by eurythmy therapy training. Evid Based Complement Alternat Med 2013;2013:564340.

37. Ong J, Sholtes D. A mindfulness-based approach to the treatment of insomnia. J Clin Psychol 2010;66:1175–84.

38. Ong JC, Shapiro SL, Manber R. Combining mindfulness meditation with cognitive-behavior therapy for insomnia: a treatment-development study. Behav Ther 2008;39:171–82.

39. Ong JC, Shapiro SL, Manber R. Mindfulness meditation and cognitive behavioral therapy for insomnia: a naturalistic 12-month follow-up. Explore (NY) 2009;5:30–6.

40. Ong JC, Ulmer CS, Manber R. Improving sleep with mindfulness and acceptance: a metacognitive model of insomnia. Behav Res Ther 2012;50:651–60.

41. Bootzin RR, Stevens SJ. Adolescents, substance abuse, and the treatment of insomnia and daytime sleepiness. Clin Psychol Rev 2005;25:629–44.

42. Britton WB, Haynes PL, Fridel KW, et al. Polysomnographic and subjective profiles of sleep continuity before and after mindfulness-based cognitive therapy in partially remitted depression. Psychosom Med 2010;72:539–48.

43. Tsao JC, Zeltzer LK. Complementary and alternative medicine approaches for pediatric pain: a review of the state-of-the-science. Evid Based Complement Alternat Med 2005;2:149–59.

44. Zeltzer LK, Jay SM, Fisher DM. The management of pain associated with pediatric procedures. Pediatr Clin North Am 1989;36:941–64.

45. Thrane S. Effectiveness of integrative modalities for pain and anxiety in children and adolescents with cancer: a systematic review. J Pediatr Oncol Nurs 2013;30:320–32.

46. Lakhan SE, Schofield KL. Mindfulness-based therapies in the treatment of somatization disorders: a systematic review and meta-analysis. PLoS One 2013;8:e71834.

47. Matsumoto M, Smith JC. Progressive muscle relaxation, breathing exercises, and ABC relaxation theory. J Clin Psychol 2001;57:1551–7.

48. Lehrer PM, Woolfolk RL, Rooney AJ, et al. Progressive relaxation and meditation. A study of psychophysiological and therapeutic differences between two techniques. Behav Res Ther 1983; 21:651–62.

49. Kanitz JL, Camus ME, Seifert G. Keeping the balance—an overview of mind-body therapies in pediatric oncology. Complement Ther Med 2013; 21(Suppl 1):S20–5.

50. Haynes SN, Adams AE, West S, et al. The stimulus control paradigm in sleep-onset insomnia: a multi-method assessment. J Psychosom Res 1982;26: 333–9.

51. Morin CM, Hauri PJ, Espie CA, et al. Nonpharmacologic treatment of chronic insomnia. An American Academy of Sleep Medicine review. Sleep 1999;22:1134–56.

52. Spielman AJ, Caruso LS, Glovinsky PB. A behavioral perspective on insomnia treatment. Psychiatr Clin North Am 1987;10:541–53.

Practical Strategies for Managing Behavioral Sleep Problems in Young Children

Brett R. Kuhn, PhD, CBSM

KEYWORDS

- Sleep • Insomnia • Infant • Toddler • Children • Pediatric • Parenting • Behavior management

KEY POINTS

- Empirically based treatments for young children with bedtime refusal and frequent night-waking have been often and fully described.
- Although clinicians are encouraged to draw from an evidence-based perspective when making treatment decisions, they are sometimes faced with unique cases or unusual circumstances that require them to think "outside the box" to solve pediatric sleep problems.
- Clinicians can build on the evidence-based approaches by identifying past treatment failures, creating a sleep-compatible bedroom environment, managing the sleep-wake schedule, optimizing parent-child interactions, adding reinforcement-based strategies, and addressing daytime behaviors or skill deficits that translate to improved child sleep.

INTRODUCTION

Sleep problems are common in early childhood and can affect virtually every realm of child and family functioning. Disturbed sleep is consistently identified among the most common concerns in clinical settings for children.[1–3] Research suggests that disturbed sleep is associated with several risk factors, including mood and anxiety disorders, disruptive behavior, and academic underachievement.[4–7] Further, this condition may become chronic and potentially persist into adulthood.[8–10] The systemic impact of sleep difficulties extends beyond the health of the affected child. Parents themselves may become frustrated and fatigued, resulting in negative parent-child interactions, parental depression, and impaired family satisfaction.[11,12]

The predominant sleep disturbance in young children is characterized as an extrinsic dyssomnia involving difficulty settling to sleep and frequent nighttime awakenings. These 2 symptoms often coexist and treatments targeting one symptom often generalize to the other because the process of initiating sleep is required not just at bedtime, but following nighttime awakenings that terminate each sleep cycle.[13–15] Although the International Classification of Sleep Disorders (ICSD), 3rd edition,[16] no longer includes specific insomnia subtype categories, the concept of "behavioral insomnias of childhood" (BIC), as put forth in the ICSD, 2nd edition (**Box 1**), is clinically still a useful one. Children with behavioral insomnia of childhood: sleep-onset association type (BIC: SOA) are often described in terms such as "she's always been a poor sleeper" or "he never learned to sleep through the night." These children frequently require parental presence and/or their physical contact to fall asleep. Once formed, however, sleep-onset

Disclosures: The author has no relevant financial or competing interests related to the content of this article.
Department of Pediatrics & Psychology, Munroe-Meyer Institute for Genetics and Rehabilitation, University of Nebraska Medical Center, 985450 Nebraska Medical Center, Omaha, NE 68198-5450, USA
E-mail address: brkuhn@unmc.edu

The child shows a pattern consistent with either the sleep-onset association type or limit-setting type of insomnia described below:

A. Sleep-onset association type (BIC: SOA) includes each of the following:

   1. Falling asleep is an extended process that requires special conditions.

   2. Sleep-onset associations are highly problematic or demanding.

   3. In the absence of the associated conditions, sleep onset is significantly delayed or sleep is otherwise disrupted.

   4. Nighttime awakenings require caregiver intervention for the child to return to sleep.

B. Limit-setting type (BIC: LS) includes each of the following:

   1. The individual has difficulty initiating or maintaining sleep.

   2. The individual stalls or refuses to go to bed at an appropriate time or refuses to return to bed after a nighttime awakening.

   3. The caregiver demonstrates insufficient or inappropriate limit-setting to establish appropriate sleeping behavior in the child.

From American Academy of Sleep Medicine. The international classification of sleep disorders, second edition: diagnostic and coding manual. Westchester (IL): American Academy of Sleep Medicine; 2005. p. 23; with permission.

associations are active regardless of the time of night a child is attempting to sleep. Thus, parents of young children with BIC: SOA rarely complain about the process required to "put" the child to sleep at bedtime, but they may not appreciate having to re-create those familiar routines several times during the night by rocking, nursing, or driving the child around in a vehicle (**Fig. 1**).

Once children develop the ability to self-soothe and initiate sleep independently, the transition from the crib to sleeping in a bed frequently presents the next challenge for families. When a toddler masters the ability to crawl out of the crib, parents suddenly find themselves without their toddler "containment device." This event places pressure on parents' ability to set and enforce effective behavioral limits to get young children into bed and then keep them there. Bedtime and

naptime refusal often emerges at this stage, with frequent "curtain calls," special requests, crying, tantrums, and exiting the bedroom. Children may engage in a wide variety of refusal behaviors to delay going to bed, to secure parental presence and attention, or to avoid separation. Children's sleep can be negatively impacted when parents are unable to effectively manage bedtime refusal. Children with behavioral insomnia of childhood: limit-setting type often obtain insufficient sleep because of delayed sleep onset; however, they typically have few arousals once they finally fall asleep (see **Fig. 2**). In cases of BIC: LS, professionals must be especially careful to avoid "blaming" the parents while at the same time giving them responsibility for making necessary changes. Before making this diagnosis prematurely, clinicians are encouraged to identify additional clues that insufficient or ineffective parental limit-setting is the primary factor contributing to the child's sleep disturbance. For example,

- Inappropriately late bedtimes that greatly vary from night to night
- Children who frequently fall asleep in various locations throughout the home depending on where they may be playing or are watching TV
- Children who are routinely allowed to stay up "just a bit longer" when they repeatedly leave the bedroom after bedtime
- Parent language suggesting the "cart is leading the horse"("He won't let us..."; "He insists that we...")
- Children who go to bed cooperatively, and fall asleep more easily or rapidly for other caregivers
- Behavior problems during the day (eg, tantrums, disruptive behavior), especially if the child is well behaved for other caregivers or in other contexts (eg, day care)

ASSESSMENT

Laboratory testing, daily sleep diaries or actigraphy, and standardized rating scales all play a role in the evaluation of disordered sleep. For behaviorally based pediatric sleep problems, however, the most useful tool is a skillfully executed clinical sleep history or initial clinical interview. Until late childhood or adolescence, sleep-related complaints come from the parents rather than the child.[17] Parents serve as the primary informants of children's sleep habits and behaviors, and it is the parents who typically make the final determination of what will be done, if anything, to address those habits and behaviors. In 2-parent

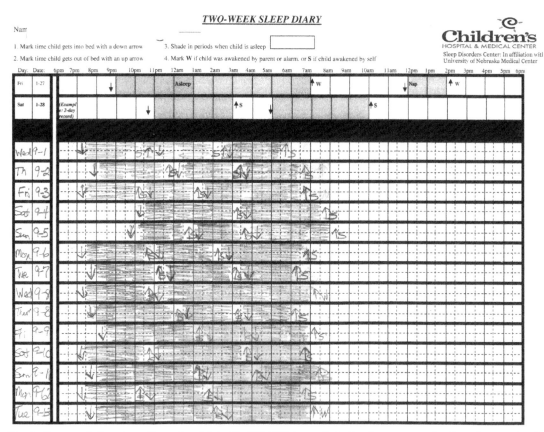

Fig. 1. Representative sleep diary of a child with BIC: SOA type. Note the frequent awakenings that tend to be brief in duration as long as a parent quickly intervenes to reestablish familiar associations and "put" the child back to sleep. (*Courtesy of* Children's Hospital and Medical Center; with permission.)

homes, it is our experience that mothers most often accompany their children to the initial sleep evaluation. Not surprisingly, spouses often have different perspectives that should not be overlooked during the evaluation. Encouraging both parents to attend is especially important when evaluating presenting problems, collaboratively determining treatment goals, and agreeing on a course of treatment.

Approaches to evaluating pediatric sleep disorders have been thoroughly described in the literature.[18,19] Our clinic implements a semistructured interview that begins with an open-ended question (eg, "what brings you in to see us today?") to get the parent and child talking.[20] Once the family is finished telling their story, the clinician follows-up with additional questions to obtain information about general health and development, past treatment attempts, and helps the family set individualized treatment goals. Sleep diaries are very useful in providing a night-by-night account of sleep, as opposed to caregiver recall, which tends to focus on global impression, the most recent nights, or the most

problematic nights. An example of a representative sleep diary for patients with BIC: SOA is shown in **Fig. 1** and BIC: LS is shown in **Fig. 2**.

The clinician then works with the family to identify potential problems across 4 major dimensions to identify modifiable factors that routinely impair sleep in children and adolescents:

- Sleep environment (light, noise, temperature, stimulation, perceived safety), including the child's ability to initiate and reinitiate sleep in this environment
- Sleep-wake schedule (supplemented by the sleep diary), including weekdays and weekends
- Parent-child interactions (during bedtime and in response to nighttime awakenings)
- Daytime problems that may impact sleep (pain; chronic medical conditions; psychiatric disorders, such as attention-deficit/hyperactivity disorder [ADHD], autism, oppositional defiant disorder [ODD]; fears/anxieties; feeding habits; medications)

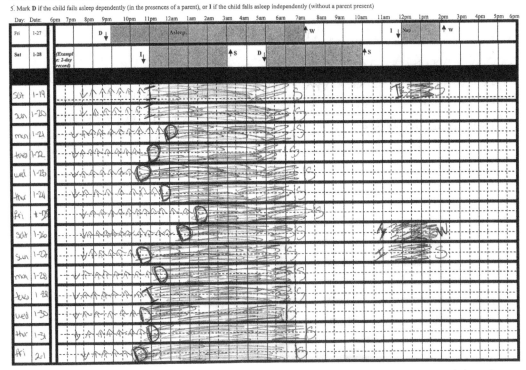

Fig. 2. Representative sleep diary of a child with BIC: LS type. Note the numerous "up and down" arrows at bedtime, indicating the child getting in/out of bed frequently, with significantly delayed sleep onset. In contrast to BIC: SOA type, children with LS type often remain asleep once they finally fall asleep because they have the ability to reinitiate sleep on waking at night without requiring parental assistance or presence. This particular child was highly persistent and successful in eventually securing parental presence at sleep onset (D, dependent sleep initiation) on 11 of 14 recorded nights despite having the skill to fall asleep independently (I, Independent sleep initiation). This "trained persistence" and unpredictable reinforcement schedule can be highly resistant to extinction-based approaches. (*Courtesy of* Children's Hospital and Medical Center; with permission.)

Taking the time to obtain a comprehensive sleep history allows the clinician to derive an *individualized, step-by-step* treatment plan and to avoid "one-size-fits-all" approaches, like handing a patient a generic list of sleep hygiene rules, or telling a parent to "just let him cry it out." Although still under the purview of evidence-based practice, generic approaches may be ineffective or inappropriate for some individuals. For example, a recently adopted 18-month-old with a history of child neglect and learned persistent responding may present an overwhelming negative response if a caregiver attempted a sudden extinction-based procedure, such as the traditional "cry-it-out" approach.

TREATMENT

Clearly, it would be preferable to prevent sleep problems from occurring in the first place rather than responding to a problem after it is firmly entrenched. Clinicians in primary care are fortunate enough to see newborn infants for whom they can practice anticipatory guidance. Common topics for anticipatory sleep guidance include ensuring safe sleep practices, initiating bedtime routines and transitional objects, regulating sleep and feeding schedules, transitioning from crib to bed, fading nighttime feedings, and encouraging parents to discuss their preferences for solitary versus co-sleeping.[21] For parents wanting their infant to sleep "through the night" the most important recommendation is to begin placing infants into their crib "drowsy but sill awake" to allow them to initiate sleep in their habitual sleep environment and set the stage for independent sleep onset. One study found that a single, 45-minute parent consultation that relied on this "drowsy but awake" principle produced infants who slept 1.3 hours more each day compared with infants in the control group.[22]

By the time most children arrive to a clinic setting, their sleep disturbance already is well established, if not well entrenched. Fortunately, the literature provides guidance for young children 5 years and younger presenting with bedtime refusal and frequent nighttime awakenings. Behavior therapy is the consensus "first-line" treatment for pediatric sleep disturbance, as studies consistently find this approach produces durable changes in more than 80% of young children.[23,24] Most empirically based sleep therapies for young children rely on extinction as the principal treatment component.[23] Widely studied options include unmodified extinction, graduated extinction, extinction with parental presence, and the bedtime pass.

Although there is a clear rational to include extinction-based procedures, it should be noted that there are some well-known inherent problems with the use of extinction. First, extinction is difficult to execute, and successful outcomes rely on a parent's ability to effectively ignore a child's disruptive bedtime behavior (sometimes for a long period). Parents may fall into the trap of selectively reinforcing novel or escalating occurrences of problem behavior, inadvertently strengthening the child's disruptive repertoire and making it more resistant to future extinction-based interventions. There are known side-effects associated with extinction, including the extinction-burst (temporary increase in frequency, duration, and/or magnitude of the behavior), which may include emotional outbursts or aggression, and spontaneous recovery (the reemergence of a problem behavior after a period of absence).[25] Parents should always be preemptively informed about the possibility of an extinction-burst. Clinicians can reframe the occurrence as a positive sign, because it means the child is aware of the change in contingency and is demonstrating a subsequent change in behavior.[26] During this stage, it is critical that parents be reassured they should stay the course because improved behavior usually is not far off.

Before implementing an extinction procedure, a thorough assessment should be conducted. By the time they are referred to a professional, many sleep-disturbed children have developed some resistance to extinction-based interventions due to a history of failed treatment attempts. Clinicians must be mindful to design a treatment approach that will address the intensity of problem behavior that may accompany children with such a history. Parents also need to be made aware that "spontaneous recovery," or the reoccurrence of a problem behavior, is more likely to occur following an environmental change (eg, travel or change of bedroom, routine, or caregiver). Again, clinicians can reframe this as a golden opportunity to enhance the flexibility and generalization of the children's sleep skills to ready them for future socialization, such as summer camps and overnight stays with friends.

Last but certainly not least, extinction may be viewed skeptically or even negatively by some parents who may find implementing such a procedure difficult or aversive. Treatment acceptability research clearly demonstrates that parents prefer "positive interventions" that rely on praise and positive reinforcement to increase adaptive skills, as opposed to interventions designed to decrease problem behavior.[27] Hence, clinicians must be prepared to present the rationale for using extinction-based interventions and discuss the specific pros and cons this intervention presents to a family.[28]

Unmodified Extinction

Extinction for pediatric sleep disturbance, also termed "sleep training," "systematic ignoring," or "the cry-it-out approach" involves having parents implement a presleep bedtime routine, placing children in bed, and ignoring all subsequent sleep-interfering behaviors (eg, crying) until morning. Parents are asked to refrain from providing attention to children except in cases of illness, danger of harm, or property destruction. Procedurally, extinction is easily understood by parents. Extinction, hereafter referred to as Unmodified Extinction (Unmodified Ext), for pediatric sleep disorders has strong grounding in learning theory. Conceptually, the acquisition of sleep-related problem behaviors (eg, bedtime tantrums, dawdling) occurs through classical or operant conditioning, and is maintained through positive and/or negative reinforcement. Negative reinforcement may occur when inappropriate behavior results in the removal (escape, avoidance) of an unpleasant event (eg, bedtime separation from parents). Problems may be positively reinforced if a preferred event occurs in response to a behavior (eg, parent physical affection in response to crying). Unmodified Ext simply involves the removal of a reinforcement contingency maintaining a response, which in turn, reduces the occurrence of that response over time. The beneficial effects of Unmodified Ext have been clearly demonstrated, earning qualification as a "well-established" intervention for bedtime disturbance and frequent night waking.[23] Unmodified Ext has been subjected to more empiric investigations, and is second in research support only to early intervention/parent education. Unmodified Ext boasts an impressive treatment effect size[29] and provides timely relief to sleep-deprived families who desire to have most crying behind them in approximately 3 nights.[28]

Graduated Extinction

As opposed to Unmodified Ext, Graduate Extinction (GE) affords parents the ability to implement planned, brief checks (eg, 15 to 60 seconds) on their child that are progressively faded. During checks, parents ensure the child's physical safety while minimizing parental attention (verbal and physical). Visits are then systematically reduced until the child initiates and maintains sleep independently. There are several variants of GE that differ in the scheduling, duration, and fading of parental check-ins. Fixed time GE uses a constant time schedule between check-ins (eg, 5 minutes), whereas "decremental" GE fades parental attention by steadily decreasing the duration of the checks themselves.[30] To illustrate, parents implementing this procedure would reduce the duration of their presence by one-seventh every 4 days over a 28-day intervention. Incremental GE, however, is by far the most commonly used approach. With incremental GE, parental checks occur on a graduated time schedule within the same night.[31] For example, parents might choose to increase the waiting time across successive checks by 5 minutes (eg, 5, 10, 15, 20 minutes). This intervention uses a paced approach that may be more desirable for parents who find Unmodified Ext too challenging to implement. However, successful use of GE relies on parents' ability to accurately and consistently deliver brief checks. Installing a video monitor in the child's bedroom allows ongoing monitoring of the child's safety, possibly reducing or eliminating the need for parents to enter the room.[32]

Extinction with Parental Presence

Extinction with parental presence (E/PP) involves following the extinction procedure (ignoring sleep-interfering child behaviors) while remaining within close physical proximity. With E/PP, parents temporarily alter their own sleeping arrangements by using a separate cot or bed within the child's bedroom. With the exception of illness, danger, or destruction of property, parents feign sleep to effectively ignore disruptive behaviors. Once the child falls asleep, parents can leave the child's bedroom to resume their typical evening activities, returning only if the child awakens. Parents continue this procedure for a specified period of time (typically 1 week) before relocating back to their own bedroom. Once out of the child's bedroom, parents are instructed to ignore the occurrence of any disruptive sleep-related behavior (Unmodified Ext). This version of extinction may offer a more gentle approach for parents and children, especially children who are heavily reliant on parent-administered sleep associations or who present with separation anxiety. Extinction with parental presence eliminates the risk of poor adherence with GE check-in procedures. There is evidence suggesting the E/PP is more effective in resolving pediatric sleep problems and results in less crying compared with Unmodified Ext and GE.[33] Moreover, this procedure may minimize the extinction burst and reduce nighttime awakenings. Treatment acceptability has not been investigated empirically, although it is plausible that some parents may be reluctant to temporarily alter their own sleeping arrangements. Also, some parents may find it more challenging to effectively ignore child distress from such close proximity. Compared with other approaches, E/PP has relatively less empiric investigation. Further research is needed to address how and when parents can transition out of the child's bedroom to avoid a spontaneous recovery of the child's disruptive bedtime behaviors.

The Bedtime Pass

The bedtime pass (BP) is a novel variant of extinction that targets bedtime resistance in children diagnosed as BIC: LS type. It is designed for slightly older (preschool to school-aged) children who have the ability to initiate sleep independently, yet resist getting ready for bed, call out from bed, or come out of the bedroom after bedtime or on awakening during the night.[34] The pass itself can be represented by any specially decorated card or object, and preferably is small enough to be placed under the child's pillow at bedtime. Parents inform the child that the pass may be exchanged for one opportunity to come out of the bedroom, or request one parent visit into the child's bedroom, after bedtime. The child is informed that once the pass is used, he or she cannot come out or call out from the bedroom again. If the child comes out of the bedroom after surrendering the pass, parents gently return the child to bed with no verbal interaction and/or attention (eg, extinction). In addition, a reward system can be implemented to motivate the child to keep the pass until morning.[35]

In sum, extinction-based interventions for bedtime refusal and frequent night-wakings are highly efficacious, but can be difficult to "sell" to some parents. Professionals may be tempted to abandon extinction-interventions in favor of more socially valid approaches. Choosing an ineffective treatment, however, is not without its own inherent risks, given the long-term negative impact of disturbed sleep on children and families.

Fortunately, there is no need to throw the baby out with the bathwater. The remainder of this article moves beyond the empirically based treatments to discuss additive and complementary interventions, along with suggestions for treatment selection, sequencing, and delivery. Readers are cautioned that many of the clinical "tricks of the trade" described have not been formally evaluated with pediatric sleep disturbance; however, most are founded on scientific principles of behavior, or in some cases are considered "proven practice" with other clinical problems of childhood.

ENHANCING EXTINCTION-BASED TREATMENTS FOR PEDIATRIC SLEEP DISTURBANCES
Identify Previous Treatment Attempts and Pinpoint Precisely Why They Were Ineffective

Before proposing an intervention plan, clinicians will want to carefully identify previous treatment attempts, including their short-term and long-term effectiveness, whether they received a sufficient trial, and any factors that accounted for their failure (eg, lack of effect, side effects, poor adherence).[36] Treatment failures with sleep-disturbed children often result from abandoning the intervention too soon because of child protests, an extinction burst, or nonadherence because parents did not agree on the course of action. Failures also occur when the bar is set too high by promising large rewards for long-term success or for behaviors that are simply beyond the child's current capabilities. A child's response to past treatment attempts may provide clues as to whether the problem represents a skill deficit ("can't do") versus performance deficit ("won't do").[37] Children who have "never slept well since birth" may be delayed in critical skill development and tend to have difficulty across contexts, even under optimal conditions. Children who possess adaptive skills, but do not use them in the desired situations, often have periods of unremarkable sleep or show complete response to incentive programs, even if short-lived.

A thorough assessment of past treatments is especially critical for families who have attempted extinction or check-in procedures. Allowing parents to occasionally "check in" on the child during extinction programs has been touted to be more "family friendly" than Unmodified Ext. The manner in which check-ins are executed, however, can be critical to the success or failure of the program. Increasing the "reinforcement value" during parental check-ins (soothing, shushing, removing child from the crib) can shape longer and longer bouts of crying. Parents who "check-in" as a response to disruptive child behavior rather than

the prescribed time schedule, risk selectively reinforcing unique or severe forms of behavior, such with as a shrill scream, a gag or gurgle, or even vomiting. One can certainly see how the execution of checking-based extinction procedures could unintentionally produce more crying and child distress, and be less "friendly" in the long-run than Unmodified Ext.

Another common treatment pitfall is the failure to "keep your eye on the prize." Independent sleep initiation is the ultimate goal for most extinction-based protocols for young children. Late termination or discontinuing extinction after a predetermined maximum duration (eg, 60 minutes) to enter the room and assist the child to sleep may produce "trained persistence" or a child who actively fights sleep. Finally, clinicians must keep in mind that extinction-based treatment failures can occur when the sleep-related problem is not maintained by the contingency purportedly being "extinguished." Ignoring repeated verbal requests will not expedite sleep onset for children placed in bed when they are not sleepy. Also, ignoring may be less effective for certain children with autism, neurobehavioral deficits, or a history of severe environmental deprivation who do not find parental presence or attention to be highly reinforcing. Thus, information obtained across the 4 critical areas of sleep (as described previously) will inform when and how an extinction-based procedure may be useful.

Provide Families a Clear Explanation of the Problem and a Rationale for the Treatment Plan

Providing parents a list of written recommendations is not sufficient. Parents require and deserve to hear the professional's conceptualization explaining why their child is not sleeping well, reasons for past treatment failures, and how the new treatment plan will overcome those problems. A thorough assessment will usually produce an idiographic treatment plan that focuses parents' efforts on addressing the significant factors contributing to the presenting problem and allow families to achieve their identified treatment goals. Parents who understand the rationale underlying their treatment approach tend to make better momentary decisions if their child throws them a "zinger" that forces them to deviate slightly from a standard protocol.

Create a Sleep-Compatible Environment and Teach the Child to Fall Asleep in That Environment

A child's habitual sleep environment, including where and with whom the child sleeps, will vary greatly depending on family values, preferences, economic status, parenting style, and cultural beliefs.[38] Designing a culturally sensitive treatment plan is more easily facilitated when families generate their own individualized treatment goals. Experts in sleep ecology have long recognized that sleep quality and duration are optimized when the sleep environment is dark, quiet, nonstimulating, and perceived to be safe.[39] Because the transition from wakefulness to sleep requires relaxation and reduced vigilance,[40,41] the presence of light and technology, especially, is associated with decreased sleep quality and quantity in children.[42,43] Young children adapt more easily to gradual modifications to their sleep environment. For example, light can be reduced by moving a lamp farther across the room or by systematically reducing the wattage of a light bulb (60, 40, 20, 7) every few nights. A bedroom television can be gradually eliminated by reducing the volume, changing to a less-preferred show, and then to an empty channel before turning it off completely. Intermittent household noises can be masked by introducing white noise, such as an electric fan, humidifier, or commercial sound screen.[44] Parents should not hesitate to make quiet, unpredictable visits to catch and praise children for "being good" in bed. These visits also allow parents to quickly identify and rectify problems in the child's bedroom, such as lights being turned on, or toys that magically find their way into a child's bed.

Optimizing the bedroom environment means little if the child falls asleep somewhere else. Children with behavioral insomnia tend to experience gross inconsistencies in their sleep environment. Their parents often wait until a child is fully asleep (and can no longer resist) before physically relocating them from the living room or parents' bedroom into the child's own bed. On awakening in the middle of the night, these children find themselves in a "foreign land" where they may have little experience initiating sleep, much less independently. Young children may attempt to avoid losing familiar sleep associations by resisting sleep onset, or insisting on physical contact with a parent to serve as a safety signal in case the parent attempts to leave once the child is asleep.

A major treatment pitfall can be averted when parents create a sleep-compatible environment and then *teach the child to fall asleep in that environment* before initiating extinction. It seems only reasonable to help facilitate more adaptive sleep associations before eliminating those that are problematic. This preparation step can be accomplished when parents require the child to fall asleep in his or her own bed, each and every time (bedtime, following nighttime awakenings,

naps). To ease the transition, parents can temporarily continue to provide the child's other familiar sleep associations (eg, singing, rubbing back, lying next to the child) to maintain cooperation and hasten sleep onset.

Select an Appropriate "Start Night"

Families may choose to immediately implement the initial steps of a treatment plan, but careful consideration should be given to selecting the "start night" for more demanding components, such as extinction. This decision should be made during a clinic visit with all of the active "players" present. Delaying treatment may be warranted in the event of stress, travel, or schedule disruptions (visitors, illness, birth of a child). In many cases, families choose to start on a night when both parents will be home and they have the weekend ahead of them (Friday night). Proving written recommendations and procedural details becomes more important when there is an anticipated delay between the clinic appointment and the selected "start night" (eg, after a vacation or holiday break).

Carefully Select Who Will Deliver the Intervention

Normally, it is a considerable advantage to have the availability of 2 parents who are both home to support each other during the introduction of treatment. This is not always the case, however. For example, we worked with a couple who mutually agreed to wait until Dad left for a business trip before starting graduated extinction. Mom was eager to get started, but Dad readily admitted that he could not tolerate even 2 minutes of listening to his daughter cry. In selected cases in which one parent routinely manages the child's sleep routines, a simple change, like switching parents, can serve as "good medicine," because certain behavior-management styles lend themselves more readily to different interventions. When considering this approach, careful consideration should be made, taking into account each parent's unique skill set and parenting style, to provide the best "fit" before determining who will deliver the intervention. For example, during the first few nights of extinction, it helps to select a parent (or a willing grandparent) who is able to enforce behavioral limits while ignoring child protests without becoming emotionally distressed or terminating the program prematurely. Once the child begins to respond to the program, the other parent can be blended back into the bedtime routine and eventually resume primary responsibility. When making this suggestion, clinicians must be careful not to blame either parent for "causing" the problem and invite parental input on who might be best suited to initiate the intervention.

Select an Appropriate Sleep-Wake Schedule and Monitor It Closely as Treatment Is Introduced

Unlike adults, young children typically do not decide when to go to bed and when to wake up. Consequently, some children may experience difficulty sleeping because of a mismatch between their inherent sleep requirement or circadian rhythm, and the sleep-wake schedule imposed on them. Parents of children with behavioral insomnias may intentionally delay their child's bedtime to avoid aversive bedtime interactions.[32] Others move their child's bedtime *earlier*, mistakenly believing that "If it takes him an hour to fall asleep, then we will start 1 hour earlier so he will be asleep by 8:30 PM." Parents who do not fully understand circadian processes find that this strategy usually backfires, making children even more resistant to the bedtime routine because they are placed in bed when they are not remotely sleepy.

To increase homeostatic sleep drive and take advantage of circadian timing, a temporary delay in the child's bedtime should be considered before implementing extinction. The objective of this step is to increase the likelihood of rapid sleep onset and (hopefully) decrease the duration of bedtime resistance. The new bedtime can be selected by adding 5 to 10 minutes to the child's average sleep onset (clock) time over the past 3 nights. Some readers may recognize this treatment component as a variation on Piazza and Fisher's highly effective bedtime fading protocol for pediatric insomnia.[45] Once the child routinely falls asleep independently within 20 to 30 minutes, the bedtime is gradually moved earlier to reach the original bedtime or the parents' bedtime goal.

Because delaying the child's bedtime increases the risk of circadian drift, morning wake-times and nap-times must be closely monitored and maintained to their pretreatment times. This practice prevents children from "making-up" for lost sleep following a difficult treatment night, increasing the likelihood they will fall asleep more quickly the following evening. Programing this intervention across a child's environmental contexts is beneficial to prevent make-up sleep or extended naps from occurring at day care or during after-school programing.

Optimize Parent-Child Interactions to Facilitate Sleep

Research has identified a long list of factors that adversely impact children's sleep. Obvious culprits include illness, pain, allergies, medical conditions, child temperament, and circadian preference. Among the numerous bio-psychosocial factors studied, the strongest predictor of sleep disturbance for infants and young children is parental management during bedtime and again in response to nighttime awakenings.[46] Although parental attention, physical proximity, and assistance during sleep onset may provide an effective short-term strategy to minimize child protests, this pattern predicts the persistence of sleep problems over time.[47] Children miss opportunities to develop adaptive sleep associations when parents remain with them until they fall asleep, place them in bed already asleep, feed or nurse them to sleep, and bring them into the parents' bed following nocturnal awakenings. Given their role in establishing and maintaining sleep problems in young children, it is not surprising that the treatment outcome research has focused primarily on modifying parent-child interactions to shape healthier child sleep patterns.[23,48]

Optimizing parent-child interactions requires clinicians to use "fact, act, and tact," to educate parents on the advantages and disadvantages of each approach, and help them settle on the treatment and pace (slow Vs accelerated) to provide the best "fit" given the child's temperament and family values.[28] Parents can be informed that the extinction-based variants are not necessarily distinct treatments, but can be viewed on a continuum based on the nonadaptive sleep association being targeted. Further, a child's age and development will heavily inform treatment. The sleep of infants tends to be more dependent on proximal stimuli, such as motion (rocking), skin-to-skin contact, nursing, or even contact with a mother's hair. With maturity and acquisition of motor skills, children begin to retrieve their own pacifiers or blankets and develop the ability self-soothe. Eliminating a child's nonadaptive sleep associations could certainly be accomplished in one fell swoop with Unmodified Ext, but many parents prefer to proceed more slowly. For example:

- Put an end to the conditioned association between nursing/feeding and sleep onset by scheduling the bedtime feeding slightly earlier and terminating it before sleep initiation.
- End the association between "skin-to-skin" contact and sleep onset, or of being rocked to sleep, by placing children in their crib drowsy but still awake, while still providing the child parental presence and liberal physical contact (stroking, pats).
- End the association of physical contact and sleep onset by gradually eliminating the

contact while maintaining parent proximity in the child's bedroom (eg, extinction with parental presence).

- End the association of parent proximity/presence and sleep onset through graduated extinction (leaving the room with scheduled checks).
- Eliminate the association between disruptive bedtime behaviors and parental attention through the use of unmodified extinction or extinction with the bedtime pass.

Decide Whether to Target All Sleep Opportunities or Take It One Step at a Time

Parents have the option to initially implement an extinction-based intervention during bedtime, or to immediately target all sleep-onset opportunities throughout the day. Overwhelmed or sleep-deprived families may be well-advised to initially focus just on bedtime for a while before intervening with nighttime awakenings and naptimes. For some, the newly developed skills at bedtime will generalize to other sleep opportunities without needing to directly target them, resulting in a child who "sleeps through the night."[31] If parents initially target bedtime only, they should respond immediately to nighttime awakenings. Hanging bells on the parent's bedroom door will signal the child's entry and prompt parents to immediately return the child to his or her bed with minimal attention.[49] Lack of independent sleep initiation is certainly not the only reason children continue to awaken at night. Children who fall asleep in one location but awaken in another may return to the original setting to reinitiate sleep. Children who take a long time to reinitiate sleep, even in their desired sleep environment, may require adjustments to their sleep schedule. Finally, clinicians can help parents identify potential reinforcers that young children prefer over resuming sleep. A key question is "what does the child usually do on awakening?" Some children find they can covertly gain access to forbidden candy, snacks, or television. Others learn to capitalize on undivided parental attention that may be unavailable to them when siblings are awake during the day. Many simply prefer their parents' bed over their own.

Turbo-Charge Any Extinction-Based Protocol by Combining It with Reinforcement for Appropriate Behavior

Although extinction is effective in reducing problem behaviors that interfere with sleep, it does little to teach and reinforce appropriate "replacement" behaviors. Basic and applied research indicates

that adding a reinforcement component to extinction-based procedures produces more rapid and effective results, and reduces the likelihood of undesirable side effects.[50,51] Consequently, implementing extinction as the sole intervention component is rarely recommended.[52]

In contrast to procedures designed to decrease problematic sleep behavior, the Positive Routines (PR) procedure targets adaptive skills by teaching parents to use differential reinforcement for appropriate behavior (eg, calm pre-bedtime behavior, independent sleep onset).[53] First, the child's bedtime is temporarily delayed to match the child's typical sleep-onset clock time. To establish the positive routine, parents identify and implement a "chain" of 4 to 7 enjoyable and relaxing pre-bedtime activities lasting no more than 20 minutes total. These activities serve as "presleep cues" or positive sleep associations. Parents provide positive attention and praise on successful completion of each link in the "chain." A head-to-head outcome study suggests that PR may offer more immediate results with fewer side effects than graduated extinction.[54]

Positive reinforcement also can be delivered in the form of tangibles (eg, candy, toys, tickets to exchange for items), social approval (eg, hug, smile, praise), or activities (eg, reading, playing a game). For example, the Mystery Motivator uses preselected squares with hidden messages decipherable with a "developer" pen. As children color in the square, invisible ink changes color, revealing a reward. Robinson and Sheridan[55] combined a Mystery Motivator and behavioral contracting to reduce bedtime noncompliance. The Sleep Fairy is another example of positive reinforcement that combines a bedtime social story with tangible rewards. The book tells a tale in which the "Sleep Fairy" leaves a small tangible reward under children's pillow at night when children exhibit appropriate sleep behaviors (eg, remaining in bed/bedroom). Research using this system demonstrated a rapid, observable decrease in disruptive bedtime behaviors.[56] Children who have outgrown the "magical" stage can still participate in positive reinforcement by developing a Grab Bag incentive system. Parents help their child develop a variety of rewards that are written on slips of paper and placed into a container. Children pick a random prize from a container immediately after demonstrating desired behavior (eg, sleep in your own bed all night).

For toddlers and preschool children, delayed delivery of tangible items will rarely compete with the immediacy and saliency of parental presence and attention. The Excuse-Me Drill (EMD) was specifically designed to reduce bedtime problems and frequent nighttime awakenings in younger children. The procedure combines the complementary forces of extinction and reinforcement to target the key skill of independent sleep initiation. The beauty of the EMD protocol is that it relies on parent behaviors that are already known to be reinforcing to the child (their own presence and attention). By simply reversing the contingency, parents deliver these social reinforcers to shape appropriate in-bed behavior rather than in response to inappropriate behavior. On completing the normal bedtime routine, the parent places the child in bed and says, "Excuse me, I need to go … [insert reason] …, but I will be right back to check on you." On the first trip, the parent barely crosses the threshold of the bedroom and (before the child has the opportunity to misbehave) quickly returns to the child to provide physical presence, attention, a calm touch, and labeled verbal praise for being a "big girl" and "staying quietly in your bed." All aspects of the reinforcement schedule, including the duration of visits, the reward "value" of parent behavior during visits, and the distance/duration away from the bedroom during excuseme trips, start on a thick schedule but are gradually faded over subsequent nights as the child develops increased behavioral mastery.

At this time, there are no controlled, large group studies demonstrating the efficacy of the EMD with sleep-disturbed children. The EMD has been described in one national conference presentation[57] and it served as the primary treatment component in a sleep intervention package for children with Angelman Syndrome.[58] Empirically based clinicians may derive some comfort, however, in knowing that the EMD simply represents the clinical application of proven, fundamental principles of behavior. Numerous intervention studies have used various forms of reinforcement and Ext to address commonly occurring as well as novel behavior problems in both children and adults. There is solid evidence that problem behavior responds more readily, with fewer side effects, when extinction and reinforcement are combined, versus using either as the sole intervention component.[51,52,59,60]

Create a Back-Up Plan for Exiting the Bedroom

Even a carefully crafted treatment plan can be challenged when children escape the bedroom and enter the living area. This behavior is less common when reinforcement is provided for appropriate in-bed behavior, but it can pose a major problem until children figure out the new program. One option is for parents to immediately return young children to their bedroom, stating firmly "it is bedtime" or "get back in bed," while minimizing eye contact and attention. On returning the child to the bedroom, a single warning can be provided: "If you come out of the bedroom again I will have to close your door." Before attempting to secure young children in a room, parents first must make sure to prepare the room by removing breakable items or furniture (mirrors, unsecured dressers) that might result in harm during a tantrum or destructive behavior. If parents are not comfortable closing the child's bedroom door, other options may be used to secure the child safely in the room, such as installing a mesh security gate at the threshold of the bedroom. Once secured, the parent remains quietly in the hallway, ignoring inappropriate behavior until the child self-calms. On 3 to 5 seconds of quiet behavior, the parent immediately opens the door or removes the gate, enters the room, and if necessary places the child back in bed before reinitiating the behavioral treatment plan. Using tangible rewards or adding the Bedtime Pass to the treatment plan may be more appropriate for older children of larger stature who repeatedly exit the bedroom.

Target Daytime Behavior and Skills That Translate to Improved Sleep

Even when sleep disturbance is the presenting concern, astute clinicians do not ignore behaviors, skill repertoires, and parent-child interactions that occur *during the day*. Although sleep disturbances certainly occur in the context of severe psychiatric disorders,[61] the most common culprits in young children involve incomplete skill attainment, poor habits, or problematic parent-child interactions. When targeted for intervention during the day, improvements in these areas can generalize to successful bedtimes and undisturbed sleep. Skill attainment can be viewed within a transactional developmental perspective. Newborns have few skills and rely largely on the parent for feeding, soothing, and helping them initiate sleep. Throughout the unfolding of development, however, children learn new skills and become more flexible and independent as parents fade their assistance and gradually turn over responsibility to the adolescent or young adult.

By inquiring about a child's daytime skills and behaviors, clinicians can gain a better idea of whether the child's sleep disturbance may be related to a child (or parent) skill-deficit or performance deficit. For example, if a child happily separates from a parent to attend day care, then problems separating at bedtime more likely reflect a failure to perform these skills under bedtime conditions, as opposed to a global skill deficit or anxiety state. Parents may be more willing to set limits at bedtime if clinicians help them recognize that their child is perfectly capable of displaying a behavior based on his or her daytime performance. On the other hand, if a child displays a true skill deficit that manifests itself throughout the day, it would seem more reasonable to build these skills slowly *during the day* before subjecting the child to an extinction-based intervention. Few parents have successfully toilet trained their child by ignoring what they DON'T want their child to do.

Feeding schedule

As mentioned earlier, clinicians will want to inquire about feeding habits both during the day and night. Infants who consume large quantities of milk at night may have developed conditioned hunger cues that trigger frequent nighttime awakenings.[62] This pattern is more common in infants who are nursed frequently throughout the day or who are given a bottle whenever they show minor signals of discomfort.[63] Intervention involves substituting other caregiving responses (eg, diapering, swaddling, rocking) to gradually lengthening feeding intervals *during the day* before phasing out the nighttime feedings.[64]

Child self-quieting skills and parental tolerance for child discomfort

Infants begin to acquire self-soothing and self-entertainment skills as they naturally become less reliant on others to entertain them and calm them whenever they get upset. For infants, these skills may involve playing with their own fingers, batting at a mobile, retrieving a pacifier, or sucking a thumb. Self-soothing skills emerge between 3 and 6 months of age for most healthy, typically developing infants, and delays in the acquisition these skills is linked to disturbed sleep.[65–67] Attempting an extinction-based intervention for young children with poor self-soothing skills may result in vomiting during the initial stages of treatment and cause parents to quickly abandon the intervention. Once again, practical parenting strategies can be used *during the day* to shape age-appropriate self-quieting skills, and to later increase a toddler's independent play skills.[68]

In some cases it is the parents, rather than the child, who require further skill development. Parents differ greatly in their tolerance for child protests (ie, whining, crying). For some, a few minutes of listening to an infant crying seems like hours, whereas other parents expertly ignore a toddler temper tantrum for 30 minutes. A parent's underdeveloped tolerance for minor forms of child discomfort may explain why sleep disturbance is

seen more frequently in first-born children.[11,69] Parents who are quick to anger may benefit from learning how to effectively ignore, or calmly return a child to the child's bedroom to avoid increased physiologic arousal. Clinicians can ask parents to provide an honest appraisal (informal rating on a 1–10-point scale) of the degree of distress they experience when their child whines, screams, or cries out. Parents can be directly taught self-regulation skills to become less hyperreactive to mild forms of child discomfort.[70] Most parents simply benefit from seeing the "other side" of a temper tantrum. Day Correction of Bedtime Problems targets critical skills that are needed by children and parents during the day and night.[71] Specifically, this procedure involves placing young children in time-out for misbehavior (eg, tantrums, aggression, refusing to accept "no" for an answer). Rather than terminating time-out after a specific time period (eg, 3 minutes), children are released on displaying self-quieting skills. Initially they are removed from time-out after 2 to 3 seconds of quiet behavior, but this criterion can be gradually increased to approximately 30 seconds of quiet before placing them back into a reinforcing "time-in" environment where parents deliver positive attention for appropriate behavior. Although the procedure teaches young children critical self-regulation skills, it also teaches parents to use ignoring and differential attention as a behavior management tool, and provides them daytime exposure to increase their tolerance to child protests.[72] Some parents need to experience the positive outcomes from successfully enforcing behavioral limits throughout the day before implementing an extinction-based protocol at bedtime.

Parental limit setting and child compliance

For young children, the phrase, "it's time for bed" triggers a stream of behavior that may include requests for more stories, drink(s) of water, acute adjustments to the lighting environment, numerous hugs and kisses, and a sudden interest in the fine art of philosophic debate. Parents unable (or unwilling) to say "no" and to enforce behavioral limits will find themselves engulfed in increasingly longer and more complex bedtime routines.[73] By the time the family reaches the clinic, a parent may sheepishly admit to hand delivering crushed ice (shaken, not stirred) with the child's fifth drink of bottled water.

Ineffective parenting is certainly not the only factor in cases presenting with BIC: Limit-Setting Type. Sometimes, the sleep environment itself contributes to difficulty setting limits, such as when child protests (eg, loud screaming, crying) interfere with the sleep of others sharing a bedroom (siblings), house (grandparents), or apartment complex (neighbors). Children with strong-willed temperaments, ODD, or ADHD, can turn minor parent requests into major power struggles. These struggles are likely to occur not just during bedtime, but during the morning routine, mealtimes, chore completion, and public outings (eg, stores).

Fortunately, there exists a strong, evidenced-based treatment for noncompliant, disruptive, and aggressive children.[74] Behavioral parent training programs (BPT) allow parents to become "co-therapists" in the treatment of their children's behavior problems. Parents receive active coaching to increase specialized skills, such as clear and effective delivery of instructions, praise, positive attention, administration of rewards and privileges, rule-setting, ignoring, reprimands, withdrawal of privileges, and time-out (a form of extinction).[75–78] BPT programs often use a (bed) room enforcement procedure, secured by a partition or door, for children who refuse to enter or remain in time-out.[76,79] A short course of behavioral parenting training to address noncompliant and defiant child behavior *during the day* may be "just what the doctor ordered" before targeting disruptive bedtime or nighttime behavior. This may be especially helpful for parents who are hesitant to use extinction-based treatments for disruptive bedtime behavior, or to use a gate door to secure young children who repeatedly refuse to remain in their bedroom.

Fear and anxiety

A large study examining sleep in children and adolescents with anxiety disorders found that 88% had at least one sleep-related problem, with the most common disturbances being insomnia, nightmares, and reluctance/refusal to sleep alone[80] (also see the article by Alfano elsewhere in this issue). Children with sleep problems are, in turn, likely to have comorbid anxieties and fears.[81]

Separation anxiety disorder (SAD) involves developmentally inappropriate and excessive fear or anxiety concerning separation from those to whom the individual is attached.[82] For many children, bedtime necessitates separation from the parent(s).[83] It should not be surprising that difficulty sleeping alone is cited as a top reason for referral to SAD treatment clinics.[84] Another common problem in young children with disturbed sleep is fear of the dark.[85] In fact, one prominent anxiety expert indicated that darkness is the 4-year-old child's single-most predominant fear.[86] We frequently encounter parents who report that their child is "scared of the dark." In our experience, most of these children sleep with a bedroom TV or overhead lights turned on for part or all of the night, which only further impairs their sleep.

There is strong consensus that exposure-based cognitive-behavioral therapy is the method of choice for anxiety disorders.[87] We frequently work with highly anxious children in our pediatric sleep clinic, using Eisen and Schaefer's[84] model of negotiating with children to gradually approach and master their own fears. For example, we may start by teaching children to cope with brief separations as a parent leaves to take a walk around the block, and work toward staying overnight at a friend's house if developmentally appropriate. Fear of the dark can be addressed by reinforcing children for tolerating increasingly darker environments over time, such as systematically reducing the bedroom light by 20 W every third or fourth night. Children can be more actively engaged through the use of graduated exposure games, such as the "blindfold game," the "toy-in-the-dark-room" game, or the "find-noisy-box-game."[85]

SUMMARY

Children with sleep disturbances frequently present with coexisting medical, neurodevelopmental, or behavioral conditions that require clinicians to enhance or alter evidence-based treatments. The primary aim of this article was to provide additional "tricks of the trade" to help practicing clinicians effectively manage behavioral sleep problems in young children. Efficacious treatments for children with disruptive behavior disorders, fears and anxieties, and sleep disturbances have many overlapping features. Optimal sequencing and integration of these treatments, however, has not yet been adequately investigated. Clinicians may choose to intervene during the day if a child displays obvious skill deficits, or when severe anxiety impairs sleep. This choice would allow gradual skill attainment at a time when children and parents are less subject to frustration and reduced willpower at day's end.[88] Children with mood disorders or disruptive behavior may be better served by first targeting the sleep disturbance, especially if the child is obtaining insufficient sleep or the occurrence of the behavior is linked to daytime sleepiness. Clues might include a predictable increase in behavior problems after missed naps or sleepless nights, behavior problems that tend to occur during a specific time of day (often late afternoon), or a child who routinely falls asleep when placed in time-out for misbehavior. Many young children obtain sufficient sleep despite lengthy bedtime struggles and frequent nighttime awakenings; therefore, parents may wish to start with a behavioral parent training program to reduce disruptive behavior throughout the day.

REFERENCES

1. Arndorfer RE, Allen KD, Aljazireh L. Behavioral health needs in pediatric medicine and the acceptability of behavioral solutions: implications for behavioral psychologists. Behav Ther 1999;30(1):137–48.
2. Keren M, Feldman R, Tyano S. Diagnoses and interactive patterns of infants referred to a community- based infant mental health clinic. J Am Acad Child Adolesc Psychiatry 2001;40(1):27–35.
3. Sinai D, Tikotzky L. Infant sleep, parental sleep and parenting stress in families of mothers on maternity leave and in families of working mothers. Infant Behav Dev 2012;35(2):179–86.
4. Gregory AM, O'Connor TG. Sleep problems in childhood: a longitudinal study of developmental change and association with behavioral problems. J Am Acad Child Adolesc Psychiatry 2002;41(8):964–71.
5. Fallone G, Owens JA, Deane J. Sleepiness in children and adolescents: clinical implications. Sleep Med Rev 2002;6(4):287–306.
6. Gruber R, Laviolette R, Deluca P, et al. Short sleep duration is associated with poor performance on IQ measures in healthy school-age children. Sleep Med 2010;11(3):289–94.
7. Lavigne JV, Arend R, Rosenbaum D, et al. Sleep and behavior problems among preschoolers. J Dev Behav Pediatr 1999;20(3):164–9.
8. Byars KC, Yolton K, Rausch J, et al. Prevalence, patterns, and persistence of sleep problems in the first 3 years of life. Pediatrics 2012;129(2):e276–84.
9. Kataria S, Swanson MS, Trevathan GE. Persistence of sleep disturbances in preschool children. J Pediatr 1987;110(4):642–6.
10. Al Mamun A, O'Callaghan F, Scott J, et al. Continuity and discontinuity of trouble sleeping behaviors from early childhood to young adulthood in a large Australian community-based-birth cohort study. Sleep Med 2012;13(10):1301–6.
11. Chi-Yung S, Sjur-Fen Gau S, Soong WT. Association between childhood sleep problems and perinatal factors, parental mental distress and behavioral problems. J Sleep Res 2006;15(1):63–73.
12. Byars KC, Yeomans-Maldonado G, Noll JG. Parental functioning and pediatric sleep disturbance: an examination of factors associated with parenting stress in children clinically referred for evaluation of insomnia. Sleep Med 2011;12(9):898–905.
13. Anders TF, Keener MA, Bowe TR, et al. A longitudinal study of night-time sleep-wake patterns in infants from birth to one year. In: Call JD, Galenson E, editors. Frontiers in infant psychiatry, vol. I. New York: Basic Books; 1985. p. 150–66.
14. Burnham MM, Goodlin-Jones BL, Gaylor EE, et al. Nighttime sleep-wake patterns and self-soothing from birth to one year of age: a longitudinal intervention study. J Child Psychol Psychiatry 2002;43(6):713–25.
15. Mindell JA. Treatment of night wakings in early childhood through generalization effects. Sleep Res 1990;19:121.
16. AASM. The international classification of sleep disorders–third edition (ICSD-3). Westchester (IL): American Academy of Sleep Medicine; 2014.
17. Ferber R. Assessment of sleep disorders in the child. In: Ferber R, Kryger M, editors. Principles and practice of sleep medicine in the child. Philadelphia: Saunders; 1995. p. 45–54.
18. Babcock DA. Evaluating sleep and sleep disorders in the pediatric primary care setting. Pediatr Clin North Am 2011;58(3):543–54.
19. Moturi S, Avis K. Assessment and treatment of common pediatric sleep disorders. Psychiatry (Edgmont) 2010;7(6):24–37.
20. Kuhn BR. Sleep disorders. In: Hersen M, Thomas JC, editors. Handbook of clinical interviewing with children. New York: Sage Publications; 2007. p. 420–47.
21. Mindell JA, Owens JA. A clinical guide to pediatric sleep: diagnosis and management of sleep problems. Philadelphia: Lippincott Williams & Wilkins; 2003.
22. Symon BG, Marley JE, Martin AJ, et al. Effect of a consultation teaching behaviour modification on sleep performance in infants: a randomised controlled trial. Med J Aust 2005;182(5):215–8.
23. Mindell JA, Kuhn B, Lewin DS, et al. Behavioral treatment of bedtime problems and night wakings in infants and young children. Sleep 2006;29(10):1263–76.
24. Morgenthaler TI, Owens J, Alessi C, et al. Practice parameters for behavioral treatment of bedtime problems and night wakings in infants and young children. Sleep 2006;29(10):1277–81.
25. Iwata BA, Pace GM, Cowdery GE, et al. What makes extinction work: an analysis of procedural form and function. J Appl Behav Anal 1994;27(1):131–44.
26. Didden R, Sigafoos J, Lancioni GE. Unmodified extinction for childhood sleep disturbance. In: Perlis M, Aloia M, Kuhn BR, editors. Behavioral treatments for sleep disorders: a comprehensive primer of behavioral sleep medicine interventions. Boston: Elsevier/Academic Press; 2010. p. 257–63.

27. Reimers TM, Wacker D, Cooper LJ. Evaluation of the acceptability of treatments for children's behavioral difficulties: ratings by parents receiving services in an outpatient clinic. Child Fam Behav Ther 1991;13(2):53–71.

28. France KG. Fact, act, and tact: a three-stage approach to treating the sleep problems of infants and toddlers. Child Adolesc Psychiatr Clin N Am 1996;5(3):581–99.

29. Kuhn BR, Elliott AJ. Treatment efficacy in behavioral pediatric sleep medicine. J Psychosom Res 2003;54(6):587–97.

30. Rolider A, Van Houten R. Training parents to use extinction to eliminate nighttime crying by gradually increasing the criteria for ignoring crying. Educ Treat Children 1984;7(2):119–24.

31. Mindell JA, Durand VM. Treatment of childhood sleep disorders: generalization across disorders and effects on family members. Special issue: interventions in pediatric psychology. J Pediatr Psychol 1993;18(6):731–50.

32. Meltzer LJ. Clinical management of behavioral insomnia of childhood: treatment of bedtime problems and night wakings in young children. Behav Sleep Med 2010;8(3):172–89.

33. France KG, Blampied NM. Modifications of systematic ignoring in the management of infant sleep disturbance: efficacy and infant distress. Child Fam Behav Ther 2005;27(1):1–16.

34. Friman PC, Hoff KE, Schnoes C, et al. The bedtime pass: an approach to bedtime crying and leaving the room. Arch Pediatr Adolesc Med 1999;153(10):1027–9.

35. Schnoes CJ. The bedtime pass. In: Perlis M, Aloia M, Kuhn BR, editors. Behavioral treatments for sleep disorders: a comprehensive primer of behavioral sleep medicine interventions. Boston: Elsevier/Academic Press; 2011. p. 293–8.

36. Sateia MJ, Doghramji K, Hauri PJ, et al. Evaluation of chronic insomnia. An American Academy of Sleep Medicine review. Sleep 2000;23(2):243–308.

37. Duhon GJ, Noell GH, Witt JC, et al. Identifying academic skill and performance deficits: the experimental analysis of brief assessments of academic skills. Sch Psychol Rev 2004;33(3):429–43.

38. Jenni OG, Werner H. Cultural issues in children's sleep: a model for clinical practice. Pediatr Clin North Am 2011;58(3):755–63.

39. Siegel JM. Phylogeny and the function of REM sleep. Behav Brain Res 1995;69(1–2):29–34.

40. Dahl RE. The regulation of sleep and arousal: development and psychopathology. Dev Psychopathol 1996;8(1):3–27.

41. Lewin DS. Behavioral insomnias of childhood-limit setting and sleep onset association disorder: diagnostic issues, behavioral treatment, and future directions. In: Perlis ML, Lichstein KL, editors. Treating sleep disorders: principles and practice of behavioral sleep medicine. Hoboken (NJ): Wiley; 2003. p. 365–92.

42. Owens J, Maxim R, McGuinn M, et al. Television-viewing habits and sleep disturbance in school children. Pediatrics 1999;104(3):e27.

43. Oka Y, Suzuki S, Inoue Y. Bedtime activities, sleep environment, and sleep/wake patterns of Japanese elementary school children. Behav Sleep Med 2008;6(4):220–33.

44. Forquer LM, Johnson CM. Continuous white noise to reduce resistance going to sleep and night wakings in toddlers. Child Fam Behav Ther 2005;27(2):1–10.

45. Piazza CC, Fisher WW. Bedtime fading in the treatment of pediatric insomnia. J Behav Ther Exp Psychiatry 1991;22(1):53–6.

46. Mindell JA, Sadeh A, Kohyama J, et al. Parental behaviors and sleep outcomes in infants and toddlers: a cross-cultural comparison. Sleep Med 2010;11(4):393–9.

47. Fehlings D. Frequent night awakenings in infants and preschool children referred to a sleep disorders clinic: the role of non-adaptive sleep associations. Child Health Care 2001;30(1):43–55.

48. Owens JA. When child can't sleep, start by treating the parents. Curr Psychiatr 2006;5(3):21–2, 27–30, 35–6.

49. Moore M. Bedtime problems and night wakings: treatment of behavioral insomnia of childhood. J Clin Psychol 2010;66(11):1195–204.

50. Lerman DC, Iwata BA, Wallace MD. Side effects of extinction: prevalence of bursting and aggression during the treatment of self-injurious behavior. J Appl Behav Anal 1999;32(1):1–8.

51. Petscher ES, Bailey JS. Comparing main and collateral effects of extinction and differential reinforcement of alternative behavior. Behav Modif 2008;32(4):468–88.

52. Lerman DC, Iwata BA. Developing a technology for the use of operant extinction in clinical settings: an examination of basic and applied research. J Appl Behav Anal 1996;29(3):345–82.

53. Milan MA, Mitchell ZP, Berger MI, et al. Positive routines: a rapid alternative to extinction for elimination of bedtime tantrum behavior. Child Behav Ther 1981;3(1):13–25.

54. Adams LA, Rickert VI. Reducing bedtime tantrums: comparison between positive routines and graduated extinction. Pediatrics 1989;84(5):756–61.

55. Robinson KE, Sheridan SM. Using the mystery motivator to improve child bedtime compliance. Child Fam Behav Ther 2000;22(1):29–49.

56. Burke RV, Kuhn BR, Peterson JL. Brief report: a "storybook" ending to children's bedtime problems—the use of a rewarding social story to reduce

bedtime resistance and frequent night waking. J Pediatr Psychol 2004;29(5):389–96.

57. Kuhn BR, Floress MT, Newcomb TC. Strategic attention for children's sleep-compatible behaviors: treatment outcome and acceptability of the "excuse-me drill". Orlando (FL): Association for Behavioral and Cognitive Therapies; November 2008.

58. Allen KD, Kuhn BR, DeHaai KA, et al. Evaluation of a behavioral treatment package to reduce sleep problems in children with Angelman syndrome. Res Dev Disabil 2013;34(1):676–86.

59. Grow LL, Kelley ME, Roane HS, et al. Utility of extinction-induced response variability for the selection of mands. J Appl Behav Anal 2008;41(1): 15–24.

60. Waters MB, Lerman DC, Hovanetz AN. Separate and combined effects of visual schedules and extinction plus differential reinforcement on problem behavior occasioned by transitions. J Appl Behav Anal 2009;42(2):309–13.

61. Ivanenko A, Barnes ME, Crabtree VM, et al. Psychiatric symptoms in children with insomnia referred to a pediatric sleep medicine center. Sleep Med 2004;5(3):253–9.

62. Ferber R. Sleeplessness in children. In: Ferber R, Kryger M, editors. Principles and practice of sleep medicine in the child. Philadelphia: Saunders; 1995. p. 79–89.

63. Elias MF, Nicolson NA, Bora C, et al. Effect of maternal care on social and emotional behavior of infants during the first year. Paper presented at: annual meeting of the Society for Research in Child Development. Detroit (MI), April 1983.

64. Ferber R, Boyle MP. Nocturnal fluid intake: a cause of, not treatment for, sleep disruption in infants and toddlers. Sleep Res 1983;12:243.

65. Sadeh A, Mindell JA, Luedtke K, et al. Sleep and sleep ecology in the first 3 years: a web-based study. J Sleep Res 2009;18(1):60–73.

66. Mindell JA, Sadeh A, Kohyama J, et al. Parental behaviors and sleep outcomes in infants and toddlers: a cross-cultural comparison. Sleep Med 2010;11(4):393–9.

67. Goodlin-Jones BL, Burnham MM, Gaylor EE, et al. Night waking, sleep-wake organization, and self-soothing in the first year of life. J Dev Behav Pediatr 2001;22(4):226–33.

68. Christophersen ER. Pediatric compliance: A guide for the primary care physician. New York: Plenum; 1994.

69. Richman N. A community survey of characteristics of one- to two- year-olds with sleep disruptions. J Am Acad Child Psychiatry 1981;20(2):281–91.

70. Tyson PD. Biodesensitization: biofeedback-controlled systematic desensitization of the stress response to infant crying. Biofeedback Self Regul 1996;21(3):273–90.

71. Christophersen ER, Harnett McConahay K. Day correction of pediatric bedtime problems. In: Perlis M, Aloia M, Kuhn BR, editors. Behavioral treatments for sleep disorders: a comprehensive primer of behavioral sleep medicine treatment protocols. Boston: Elsevier/Academic Press; 2010. p. 311–7.

72. Edwards KJ. The use of brief time-outs during the day to reduce bedtime struggles. Diss Abstr Int 1993;54:2181.

73. Owens-Stively J, Frank N, Smith A, et al. Child temperament, parenting discipline style, and daytime behavior in childhood sleep disorders. J Dev Behav Pediatr 1997;18(5):314–21.

74. Shriver MD, Allen KD. Working with parents of noncompliant children: a guide to evidence-based parent training for practitioners and students. Washington, DC: American Psychological Association; 2008.

75. Brinkmeyer MY, Eyberg SM. Parent-child interaction therapy for oppositional children. In: Kazdin AE, Weisz JR, editors. Evidence-based psychotherapies for children and adolescents. New York: Guilford Press; 2003. p. 204–23.

76. McMahon RJ, Forehand RL. Helping the noncompliant child: family-based treatment for oppositional behavior. 2nd edition. New York: Guilford Press; 2003.

77. Patterson GR. Living with children: new methods for parents and teachers. Revised edition. Champaign (IL): Research Press; 1976.

78. Webster-Stratton C. The incredible years: a trouble-shooting guide for parents of children ages 3-8 years. Toronto (Canada): Umbrella Press; 1992.

79. McNeil CB, Hembree-Kigin TL, editors. Parent-child interaction therapy. 2nd edition. New York: Springer; 2010.

80. Alfano CA, Ginsburg GS, Kingery JN. Sleep-related problems among children and adolescents with anxiety disorders. J Am Acad Child Adolesc Psychiatry 2007;46(2):224–32.

81. Chorney DB, Detweiler MF, Morris TL, et al. The interplay of sleep disturbance, anxiety, and depression in children. J Pediatr Psychol 2008; 33(4):339–48.

82. American Psychiatric Association. Diagnostic and statistical manual of mental disorders. 5th edition. Arlington (VA): American Psychiatric Publishing; 2013.

83. Sadeh A. Cognitive-behavioral treatment for childhood sleep disorders. Clin Psychol Rev 2005; 25(5):612–28.

84. Eisen AR, Schaefer CE. Separation anxiety in children and adolescents. New York: Guilford Press; 2005.

85. Mikulas WL. Graduated exposure games to reduce children's fear of the dark. In: Perlis M, Aloia M,

Kuhn BR, editors. Behavioral treatments for sleep disorders: a comprehensive primer of behavioral sleep medicine treatment protocols. Boston: Elsevier/Academic Press; 2011. p. 319–23.

86. Ollendick TH. Fear reduction techniques in children. In: Hersen M, Eisler RM, Miller PM, editors. Progress in Behavior Modification, vol. 8. New York: Academic Press; 1979. p. 127–68.

87. Silverman WK, Dick-Niederhauser A. Separation anxiety disorder. In: Morris TL, March JS, editors. Anxiety disorders in children and adolescents. 2nd edition. New York: Guilford Press; 2004. p. 164–88.

88. Teitelbaum P. Levels of integration of the operant. In: Honig WK, Staddon JER, editors. Handbook of operant behavior. (NJ): Prentice Hall; 1977. p. 7–27.

Assessment and Treatment of Delayed Sleep Phase Disorder in Adolescents
Recent Innovations and Cautions

Michael Gradisar, PhD[a],*, Marcel G. Smits, MD, PhD[b],
Bjørn Bjorvatn, MD, PhD[c]

KEYWORDS

- Delayed sleep phase disorder • Delayed sleep phase syndrome • Adolescence
- Daytime sleepiness • Sleep-onset latency • Melatonin • Dim-light melatonin onset
- Bright-light therapy

KEY POINTS

- Delayed sleep phase disorder (DSPD) is prevalent in sleep-disordered adolescents seeking treatment; its consequences include comorbid affective, academic, and behavioral dysfunction.
- Diagnosis of DSPD includes sleep monitoring (diary, actigraphy) and clinical sleep history interview, although a clinical assessment of dim-light melatonin onset is also possible. Polysomnography and questionnaires can offer additional and valuable information.
- Bright-light therapy and pharmaceutical melatonin are the most validated and clinically effective treatments for adolescents with DSPD. Novel portable light-emitting diode devices can now be used for bright-light therapy.
- Clinicians should exercise caution with the use of prolonged-release melatonin (eg, Circadin) and chronotherapy for adolescents experiencing DSPD.

INTRODUCTION

There have been many reviews and articles that fully or partly describe the treatment of delayed sleep phase disorder (DSPD),[1–5] including articles in this journal[6] and by the authors.[7,8] Therefore, a challenge is presented: what can this article bring forth that is unique to this topic? First, most of the previous literature has been tailored primarily to young adults, so the focus herein is on adolescents living in the "iEra" and the subjective experience of the adolescent with DSPD. Second, new assessment methods of circadian misalignment, in addition to new medications and devices intended to advance sleep timing, are now available, and these are discussed. Finally, preliminary evidence for the use of psychological therapies to augment classic chronobiological treatments for DSPD is presented.

Funding Sources: Nil.
Conflict of Interest: Received partial project funding from Re-Time Pty Ltd (M. Gradisar); Nil (M.G. Smits, B. Bjorvatn).
[a] School of Psychology, Flinders University, GPO Box 2100, Adelaide, South Australia 5001, Australia; [b] Department of Neurology, Hospital Gelderse Vallei, Centre for Sleep-Wake Disorders and Chronobiology, Willy Brandtlaan 10, Ede, 6716 RP, The Netherlands; [c] Department of Global Public Health and Primary Care, Norwegian Competence Center for Sleep Disorders, Haukeland University Hospital, University of Bergen, Jonas Lies vei 65, Bergen 5021, Norway
* Correspondence author.
E-mail address: grad0011@flinders.edu.au

"WHY CAN'T I SLEEP?… LEAVE ME ALONE, I JUST WANT TO SLEEP-IN"

Various descriptions of DSPD have been provided in the literature,[5,9] but few from the adolescents' perspective.[10] Over the course of adolescent development, a tendency for sleep timing to gradually delay becomes evident, with the onset often occurring around the time of pubertal development rather than being linked to chronologic age.[1,11] With increasing autonomy and relaxed parent-set bedtimes on weekends,[12,13] adolescents typically go to bed later on weekend nights (Friday and Saturday).[1,11] When weekend morning commitments are lacking, there is potential for the adolescent to "sleep-in" (**Fig. 1**, We [in red]). A weekend of sleeping-in can delay adolescents' circadian rhythm timing by as much as 1.5 hours.[14] A late rise time on Sunday means sleep homeostatic pressure has less time to accumulate and fails to peak by parents' prescribed Sunday-night bedtime,[13,15] leading to difficulty initiating sleep (see **Fig. 1**, B and S [in red]). School-night sleep is further restricted when the adolescent has to rise early for school (see **Fig. 1**, Wd [in red]), and daytime sleepiness ensues for the better part of the school morning. If this cycle persists over months, it may cause significant distress and impairment that warrants a diagnosis of DPSD.[16,17]

ASSESSMENT

Although specific protocols may vary across clinical settings, the diagnosis of DSPD in adolescents usually involves a combination of clinical interviews, sleep monitoring in the home environment, and a selection of questionnaires. Not all are needed to diagnose DSPD, but collectively they provide valuable information to inform treatment. The description given here is based largely on the authors' own clinical experience, but is also applicable to other practice settings. Before the clinic visit, adolescents and families are asked to complete sleep monitoring for at least 1 week along with a set of questionnaires, which are then used to inform and supplement the in-person clinical sleep history interview.

Misaligned Sleep Timing

Sleep diaries

Although a detailed clinical history can estimate delayed sleep timing, prospective measurement is desirable and essential for a formal diagnosis.[17] A sleep diary is a simple, validated, and inexpensive method for collection of these data (**Fig. 2**). Completion of a sleep diary over 1 week can provide evidence of (1) stable delay in sleep timing that conflicts with societal norms (eg, starting school), (2) normal sleep when free of social obligations (eg, weekends), and (3) associated sleep-onset insomnia (ie, lengthy sleep-onset latencies). Sleep diaries are less able to demonstrate difficulty in waking or daytime sleepiness, although ratings of these may be inserted into the diary at the clinician's discretion.

Actigraphy

Wrist actigraphy is another prospective measurement of sleep timing, which may complement sleep diaries. Worn like a wristwatch, an actigraph measures gross motor movement, often recorded continuously, yet with data binned into 1-minute epochs.[18,19] Accompanying software usually applies a computerized algorithm to automatically score each minute over the week as "wake" or "sleep" in the resulting actogram (**Fig. 3**). The clinician can manually select bedtimes and rise times for each night based on the sleep diary. Discrepancies between the sleep diary and actigraphy should be discussed with the adolescent (eg, actigraphy shows the adolescent is active, yet the diary shows still being asleep in bed) to ensure the validity of the data. A wrist actigraph worn on the

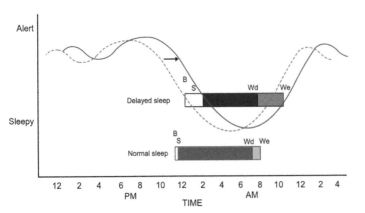

Fig. 1. The delayed circadian rhythm of alertness and sleep (*red*) relative to a normal rhythm and sleep (*blue*). B, bedtime; S, sleep onset; Wd, wake-up time on weekdays; We, wake-up time on weekends. This figure can be used in the first treatment session as psychoeducation for the adolescent.

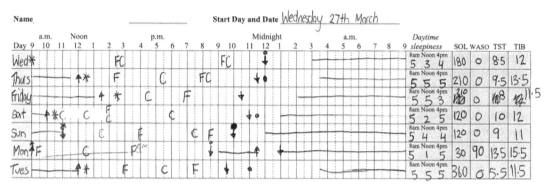

Fig. 2. Seven-day sleep diary of a 17-year-old female adolescent with delayed sleep phase disorder (DSPD). Downward arrow, bedtime; upward arrow, out of bed; circle, lights out; solid line, sleep; asterisk, first exposure to outdoor light; C, caffeinated beverage; F, meal; SOL, sleep-onset latency (minutes); WASO, wake after sleep onset (minutes); TST, total sleep time (hours); TIB, time in bed (hours); daytime sleepiness ratings (1–5), more daytime sleepiness with higher scores.

nondominant hand is recommended to assess sleep timing (ie, sleep onset and sleep offset),[20] but caution should be used in interpreting sleep-duration data. For example, male adolescents appear to move during sleep yet tend not to record this activity as wakefulness on sleep diaries.[21] Therefore, clinicians should avoid placing too much importance on sleep duration, and instead focus on sleep timing.

Polysomnography

The gold standard of sleep assessment is polysomnography (PSG). If PSG is performed according to the adolescent's habitual sleep-wake rhythm,

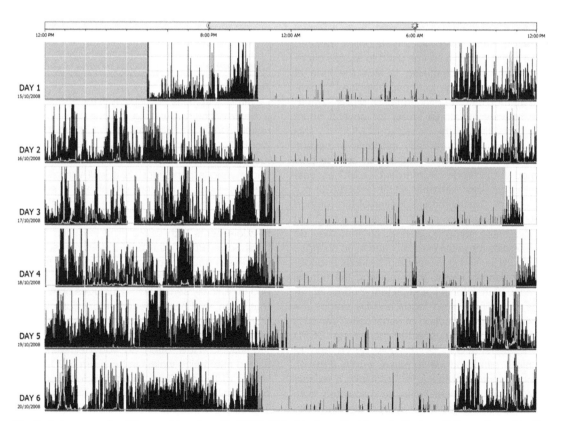

Fig. 3. Actogram of a 15-year-old male with DSPD. Thin black vertical bars indicate activity; yellow thin line indicates light intensity; blue horizontal bars are manually set based on the sleep diary's time in bed; thin red horizontal lines indicate algorithm-defined wakefulness.

the recording shows a delayed sleep period, yet with a normal distribution of sleep stages and consolidated sleep.[22] However, PSG is seldom indicated in adolescents with DSPD, in part because the diagnostic criteria for DSPD require consecutive nights of sleep monitoring, which is not feasible with PSG. PSG monitoring is generally unnecessary unless there is a clear indication of the presence of a comorbid sleep disorder such as obstructive sleep apnea (eg, snoring), periodic limb movement disorder, or narcolepsy, which may aid in the differential diagnosis of DSPD symptoms (eg, daytime sleepiness).[17]

Dim-light melatonin onset

Diagnostic criteria for DSPD specify that assessment of the patient's endogenous dim-light melatonin onset (DLMO) is "useful for confirmation of the delayed phase".[17(p119)] Melatonin is a hormone produced by the pineal gland, and the timing of its secretion is regulated by the endogenous circadian pacemaker. In entrained individuals keeping a regular sleep-wake schedule, melatonin levels are low to absent during the daytime, begin to increase in the evening, and peak during the nighttime hours. Melatonin secretion is suppressed by light,[23] so melatonin levels must be measured in dim-light conditions to accurately reflect actual secretion. Serial sampling of melatonin measured in the blood or saliva can be used to assess circadian timing by determining DLMO, the time at which levels increase to above baseline.[24] A reliable method for determination of DLMO is to measure salivary melatonin levels for several hours around the time of the expected DLMO.[25–27] This assay is now commercially available in several countries for clinical purposes, and can be performed in the home environment. DLMO assessment costs approximately €150 (~US$200) per adolescent. Crucial to the success of this method is (1) that subjects remain in dim lighting (<30 lux) for the entire sampling period, (2) that they do not exercise (physical exercise, and even changes in posture [ie, sitting to standing] reduces endogenous melatonin levels, thus masking the natural increase of melatonin.), and (3) that modest limitations regarding certain foods and beverages are applied. Hourly collection of serial saliva samples from adolescents suspected of having DSPD (13–18 years) at 8 PM, 9 PM, 10 PM, 11 PM, and 12 midnight can produce a partial curve (**Fig. 4**), which in most individuals[26,28] provides a reliable DLMO estimate. DLMO can be calculated from the serial samples by linear interpolation between adjacent points, looking for the time at which rising melatonin levels cross a predetermined threshold. Nagtegaal and colleagues[29] recommended a fixed

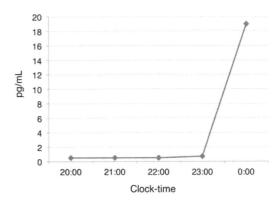

Fig. 4. Partial melatonin curve of a female adolescent, aged 15 years, falling asleep at approximately 3:30 AM and waking up without an alarm clock at approximately 4 PM.

threshold of 4 pg/mL in saliva, whereas others have suggested a threshold of 3 pg/mL to determine DLMO from saliva.[28,30]

Clinicians who require objective verification of sleep phase in their adolescent patients (eg, because of uncertainty with subjective reports) and for whom a home assay is available should consider salivary DLMO assessment. The adolescent's DLMO estimate can then be used to develop a tailored evening melatonin treatment plan (see later discussion on melatonin treatment).

Questionnaires

Daytime sleepiness

Daytime sleepiness, particularly in the morning with extreme difficulty in waking, is a common symptom resulting from circadian misalignment.[17,31] The Epworth Sleepiness Scale (ESS), which asks the respondent to rate the likelihood of falling asleep under various conditions, is a well-validated tool used to measure daytime sleepiness in adults.[32] Though clinically sensitive to treatment effects in adults,[33] the ESS may underestimate sleepiness in adolescents with DSPD. The Pediatric Sleepiness Scale (PDSS) is a brief 8-item measure that possesses good psychometric properties for children and adolescents aged 8 to 15 years,[31,34,35] and is clinically sensitive.[31] It includes many items that align well with the common complaint in DSPD of increased morning sleepiness (eg, "How often do you have trouble getting out of bed in the morning?", "How often do you decrease back asleep after being woken in the morning?"). Cutoff scores of 15 and 20 are recommended in community samples[35] and clinical samples,[34] respectively. The 20-item Chronic Sleep Reduction Questionnaire (CSRQ)[36,37] measures different symptoms of chronic sleep loss, including Shortness of sleep (6 items; eg, "I am a person who does not get enough sleep"), Sleepiness (4 items; eg, "Do you feel sleepy during the day?"), Loss of energy (5 items; eg, "I am active during the day"), and Irritability (5 items; eg, "Others think that I am easily irritated"). Adolescents with DSPD score significantly higher on the CSRQ in comparison with adolescents from the general population (van Maanen A, Dewald-Kaufmann JF, Oort FJ, et al, 2014. Screening for sleep reduction in adolescents through self-report: development and validation of the Sleep Reduction Screening Questionnaire [SRSQ]). The CSRQ also demonstrates good clinical sensitivity; for example, decreases in CSRQ scores occur following melatonin treatment for DSPD.[38]

Clinical Sleep History Interview

Ideally, the adolescent will present to the clinic with a completed sleep diary and questionnaires, in addition to data from actigraphy, PSG, and/or DLMO assessment(s) as indicated. The clinical sleep history interview is designed to supplement these data, with a focus on information not easily captured by diaries and questionnaires (eg, difficulty falling asleep at conventional times but little trouble at later times, significant disruption to life owing to the sleep disorder, extent to which sleep disruption affects school attendance/performance), as well as other information that will help to inform treatment.

The predominant complaints by adolescents with DSPD include sleep-onset insomnia, oversleeping/daytime sleepiness, and poor school attendance.[10,31] It is imperative that the clinician confirms that the cause of these symptoms results from circadian misalignment. For example, sleep-onset insomnia may result from conditioned insomnia without circadian misalignment, in which case psychophysiologic insomnia may be the most appropriate diagnosis.[17] One key differentiating factor is the extent to which the adolescent sleeps-in on weekends or oversleeps on weekdays,

which in turn interferes with school attendance (**Fig. 5**). An adolescent with an insomnia disorder may sleep later on weekends, but usually by only a small amount compared with school-day wake times. Other questions that may help to identify a circadian component of the adolescent's sleep-onset insomnia are shown in **Fig. 5**.

Other sleep disorders such as behaviorally induced insufficient sleep syndrome (BIISS), various forms of hypersomnia, and sleep-related breathing disorders all include daytime sleepiness as central to their constellation of symptoms[17] and should be part of the differential diagnosis of DSPD. The following are important clinical differentiating factors. (1) Adolescents with BIISS have restricted their sleep opportunity over time, thus producing significant sleepiness. However, they are unlikely to have difficulty falling asleep when attempting this at an earlier time. (2) Similarly, patients with hypersomnia of varying etiology would have little difficulty falling asleep. (3) Patients with symptoms of (snoring, breathing pauses) and risk factors for sleep-disordered breathing (family history, overweight) often exhibit daytime sleepiness manifestations, although these are not usually accompanied by significant sleep-onset delay.

It is also important to screen for comorbid mental, medical, and neurologic conditions, and for use of substances and prescribed medications, both as part of the differential diagnosis of prolonged sleep-onset latency and daytime sleepiness and because these may affect adherence to treatment. However, in the authors' experience most comorbid conditions have not systematically affected treatment outcomes.

In some instances, the presence of comorbid conditions may help guide the choice of treatment. For example, major depressive disorder is a common comorbid condition with DSPD, but treatment targeted toward sleep problems can still be successful. Some adolescents may exhibit light sensitivity that results in headaches, nausea, and

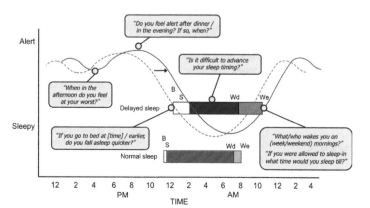

Fig. 5. Questions to ask in the clinical sleep history interview to assist in differentiating DSPD from other sleep disorders with significant sleep-onset insomnia and/or daytime sleepiness. B, bedtime; S, sleep onset; Wd, wake-up time on weekdays; We, wake-up time on weekends.

migraines, or have risk factors for the sequelae from light therapy, such as exacerbation of bipolar disorder. These caveats may suggest that selection of particular treatment strategies (eg, bright-light therapy) should be avoided. Finally, it should also be noted that internet use disorder is now included in the 5th edition of the *Diagnostic and Statistical Manual of Mental Disorders*[16]; as a likely common comorbid condition with DSPD, this combination may prove to be one of the most significant challenges in the treatment of DSPD in future years.

Other questions that may be included in the clinical interview include items targeting difficulties experienced in previous attempts to advance sleep timing, the extent of technology use (ie, screens/monitors) close to bedtime, previous treatment strategies used (including medications) and their outcomes, and the adolescent's treatment goals (eg, fall asleep quicker/earlier, return to school).

A final key point regarding assessment involves the importance of ascertaining other factors that could potentially interfere with adherence to and success of treatment. The term motivated DSPD has been used to describe patients for whom maintenance of symptoms may be associated with a secondary gain; this is particularly a concern with adolescents who have sporadic school attendance or have ceased attending altogether. For example, an adolescent with DSPD may be socially anxious and/or have a learning disability associated with poor school performance.[31] Reinitiating social contact and catching up on school work can be anxiety-provoking stimuli. In the authors' experience, these types of situations present a significant barrier to successful outcomes and may require more intensive intervention (see later discussion on motivational interviewing).

Assessment of DSPD in adolescents: Key points	
For Diagnosis	**Nondiagnostic Tools**
Clinical sleep history interview	Polysomnography
7-day sleep diary	Pediatric Daytime Sleepiness Scale
Wrist actigraphy	Chronic Sleep Reduction Questionnaire— Short Form
Dim-light melatonin onset	

TREATMENTS FOR DSPD IN ADOLESCENTS
Bright-Light Therapy

Treatment of DSPD with bright light is phase dependent. Laboratory studies have demonstrated that light administered before core temperature minimum causes phase delays, whereas light administered afterward produces phase advances.[5,7] A noninvasive and affordable technique that clinicians may use to assess the circadian rhythm of core temperature in adolescents with DSPD is as yet unknown. Although this does pose a challenge in terms of timing of light exposure, the authors have developed a protocol (detailed here) for delivery of bright-light therapy, which seems to be clinically effective and well tolerated.

Bright-light therapy, using either broad-spectrum light from specialized lamps (1000–10,000 lux), or (weather permitting) natural sunlight, can be effective in advancing an adolescent's sleep timing.[31,33,39] The sensitive period of the phase-advancing portion of the light phase-response curve (PRC) is near adolescents' natural wake-up time.[7] Clinicians are encouraged to explain this sensitive period to adolescents and parents, as the adolescent will need to sleep until their natural wake-up time on Day 1 of bright-light therapy (eg, 12 noon). Sleeping-in will appeal to adolescents, but seems counterintuitive to uninformed parents. Each successive day of treatment, the adolescent rises 30 to 60 minutes earlier (Day 2, 11 AM; Day 3, 10 AM; and so forth) and is exposed to bright light.[33,39] Wake-up time is advanced until the desired sleep-onset and -offset times are reached, which usually takes 1 to 2 weeks, depending on the severity of the circadian delay. In the authors' experience, 60-minute advances in rise time per day are workable the first few days, but as rise time advances this becomes more difficult (around 9 AM). Adolescents may then switch to 30-minute advanced rise times each day[31,33,39] until they reach a target of approximately 6 to 7 AM, at which point their sleep timing is usually "normal."[31]

Although bright-light therapy can be performed during nonschool periods, the authors have had success implementing treatment during school terms, with adolescents typically missing a few days to a week of morning classes. It is particularly important to work cooperatively with families and schools during this phase of treatment. After target sleep and wake times are reached, this sleep schedule should be strictly adhered to for at least 1 week, followed by mini-experiments of sleeping a bit later on weekends (but still within a 2-hour window of the weekday wake-up time) and/or staying up later on weekend nights. These experiments can be safely performed under supervision, and can help identify possible triggers for relapse before ceasing treatment. It is important that while performing bright-light therapy the adolescent should not be exposed to bright light in the hours before sleep onset, as this may counteract phase advances made with bright-light therapy after the sleep period. Dim light before sleep (eg, <100–150 lux), the use of tinted goggles or sunglasses, and/or limited dim screen light (ie, <1 hour)[40,41] are recommended. **Fig. 6** provides an illustration of when to provide bright light and dim light, with arrows indicating a gradual phase advancement of bright light until desired sleep timing is achieved. Recent evidence shows that the adolescent with DSPD will often need to continue to receive bright light in the morning to maintain entrained sleep timing,[33,39] but may temporarily cease treatment (eg, 1–2 weeks) to assess whether continued treatment is needed.

Light devices may be purchased at pharmacies or various agencies in many countries; however, most are not scientifically validated. In October 2012, Re-Timers, which are short-wavelength (green) light-emitting diode (LED) "glasses," were made commercially available to the public (**Fig. 7**; www.re-timers.com). These glasses were based on evidence published a decade ago[42] of significant melatonin suppression and phase change from a portable source of short-wavelength light. Preliminary testing with adolescents with DSPD has shown these to be acceptable and effective, producing clinical significant advancement of sleep timing and self-reports of improved alertness, mood, and morning behavior. However, trials comparing Re-Timers with other active treatments and control conditions are needed to validate their efficacy in adolescents with DSPD.

Bright-light treatment for DSPD in adolescents: Key points

Allow the adolescent to sleep-in, and then provide bright light

Advance rise time by 30 to 60 minutes per day, providing bright light on awakening

If advancing by 60 min/d, advance rise times by 30 min/d when wake-up time reaches ~9 AM

Treatment advancement ceases when rise time reaches 6 to 7 AM

Maintain consistent bright light for at least 1 to 2 weeks

Melatonin Treatment

Treatment of DSPD with melatonin is also phase dependent; however, its phase-changing properties are the inverse to those of bright light. That is, melatonin administered at different times can produce opposing results, potentially worsening DSPD rather than improving it. When exogenous

melatonin is administered hours before DLMO, there are phase advances of the melatonin rhythm and associated sleep timing (**Fig. 8**). However, if melatonin is instead given hours after DLMO, the rhythms are delayed (ie, sleep timing shifts later; see **Fig. 8**).[43–46] Therefore, knowledge of DLMO can be crucial to a successful treatment outcome. Two meta-analyses reported a significant decrease in sleep-onset latency when exogenous melatonin was administered according to DLMO.[47,48] This finding is in contrast to that of a different meta-analysis in which most studies administered melatonin at a time relative to bedtime. In these cases, no significant improvement of sleep was found.[49] Circadian shifts also depend on dosage,[43,48] such that high doses may maintain endogenous melatonin levels hours past DLMO, which can either delay the rhythm or cancel out phase-advancing shifts.[50] In adolescents, melatonin should be administered 4 to 5 hours before DLMO, but not earlier than 7 PM.[51] Thus, for the example in **Fig. 4** where DLMO is 12 midnight, the clinician may either suggest melatonin 5 hours beforehand (ie, 7 PM), and maintain this administration time; or 4 hours beforehand (ie, 8 PM), then gradually advance the timing (ie, 7:30 PM, then 7 PM). The starting dose is 1 mg. When the adolescent does not experience any sleep-onset advance, the dose is increased by 1 mg every week until sleep timing advances and daytime functioning improves (using the CSRQ or PDSS).[38] The maximum dose is usually 5 mg. When 1 mg advances the sleep-wake rhythm, the adolescent is advised to lower the dose until the lowest effective dose is reached.

These recommendations are based on availability of melatonin tablets produced by a compound pharmacist. A new prolonged-release formulation (Circadin), containing 2 mg of melatonin, is indicated for the short-term treatment of primary insomnia in older adults (≥55 years). It is marketed across Europe, Australasia, and parts of Asia and South America but is not yet available in the United States. As Circadin contains 2 mg of melatonin, the authors have observed cases whereby Circadin was prescribed for adolescents with DSPD before presenting to a sleep clinic. However, owing to Circadin's prolonged release of melatonin over a purported 8 to 10 hours, this not only affects the phase-advancing portion of the melatonin PRC, but has the potential to also affect the phase-delaying portion (see **Fig. 8**). Therefore, evening administration of Circadin, especially close to an adolescent's sleep-onset time, has the potential to maintain, if not worsen, the adolescent's delayed sleep timing. The authors have observed several such reports of adolescents

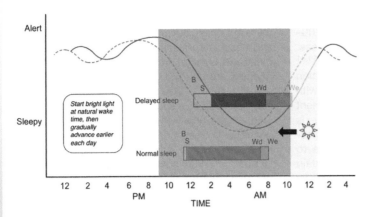

Fig. 6. When to administer evening dim light and bright light to phase-advance sleep timing. The red solid curve for delayed sleep can be representative of both sleepiness and core temperature. Bright light after core temperature nadir, phase advances sleep timing; bright light before the nadir produces phase delays, which should be avoided.

with DSPD not improving or worsening after commencement of Circadin, and therefore do not recommend the use of Circadin in the treatment of DSPD in adolescents. Furthermore, Neurim Pharmaceutical state that the "safety and efficacy of Circadin in children aged 0–18 years has not yet been established."[52]

Melatonin treatment for DSPD in adolescents: Key points

DLMO can be assessed clinically, which provides a tailored treatment program for evening melatonin administration

Melatonin tablets should begin at 1 mg per night

Provide melatonin tablets approximately 4 to 5 hours before the adolescent's DLMO

For nonresponse, increase dosage by 1 mg

Advance the administration of melatonin by 30 to 60 minutes per night

Treatment advancement ceases when sleep timing is stabilized on a low dose (eg, 1 mg)

Although this article presents bright-light therapy and melatonin administration as separate treatments, both techniques are often combined in clinical practice to phase-advance adolescents' sleep timing, and this should be considered as a treatment option.[33,39]

Chronotherapy

Whereas there is solid evidence to support the use of bright light and exogenous melatonin to treat DSPD, including in adolescents, chronotherapy as a treatment option has less empiric support.[53] Chronotherapy works by successively delaying sleep timing ("forward around the clock") until the desired sleep-onset and sleep-offset times

are achieved. Recommendations are to delay bedtime by 2 to 3 hours per day in adults.[5,53] There are several disadvantages; although chronotherapy may take the same amount of time to complete as bright light therapy, it is often more disruptive to schooling, as consecutive entire days may be missed while the adolescent is sleeping during the day. In the authors' experience, chronotherapy is also not often chosen by adolescents when given the option. Although chronotherapy is listed here as a possible option to treat DSPD in adolescents, its utility is most likely limited to situations in which the adolescent is extremely phase delayed (ie, sleep onset >4–6 AM), does not respond to bright-light therapy and melatonin treatment, and/or is already not attending school.

Motivational Interviewing to Change Sleep Behaviors

The techniques described herein can be challenging in regard of adherence for many adolescents with DSPD. Indeed some adolescents are

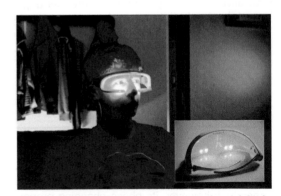

Fig. 7. Re-Timers (Re-Time Pty Ltd, Adelaide, Australia) are a new portable short-wavelength light source that can be used to phase-advance adolescents' delayed sleep patterns. (*Courtesy of* Re-Time Pty Ltd, Adelaide, Australia; with permission.)

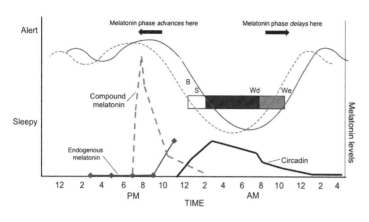

Fig. 8. Graphic illustration of when to provide melatonin tablets (*gray dashed line*), in relation to dim-light melatonin onset (final point on *red line*). Providing Circadin close to bedtime results in melatonin being released over the phase-delay portion (ie, last half of sleep period).

not aware that they have a sleep problem,[10,54] and many are unmotivated to attend sessions and drop out of treatment.[31,55] Motivational interviewing is emerging as a supplementary technique to encourage adolescents to recognize their sleep problem and regularize their behavior.[56] **Fig. 9** illustrates the various motivational stages that adolescents may present with at treatment.[57] Techniques to be used will depend on their stage of change.

In Pre-contemplation, the adolescent does not recognize that he or she has a sleep problem. Here the clinician can educate the adolescent on what constitutes a sleep problem (eg, short sleep duration, significant wakefulness in bed, significant daytime sleepiness) and potential consequences (eg, poor school performance,[58] increased risk of accidents, onset of mood and anxiety disorders). A discussion, even in the third person (eg, "What do others say about you that may suggest you're not sleeping well?"), may lead the adolescent to elicit other consequences.

From here, some adolescents may move to the Contemplation stage whereby they recognize their sleep problem, yet are unmotivated to change. The clinician is encouraged to first explore with the adolescents the advantages of their sleep pattern, and specifically the behaviors of staying up late and/or sleeping-in. The disadvantages of each behavior are explored. As adolescents state that DSPD may prevent goal attainment and distort significant others' views of them,[10] the clinician can ask how adolescents' current sleep pattern aligns with concrete goals for the future (eg, good grades, employment options, purchasing assets), in addition to their own personal values (eg, "What words would people use to describe me in the morning?", "What words would I like them to use?"). Voicing such discrepancies may arouse unsettling emotions, so the clinician is encouraged to explore positive aspects, such as how life would be different if adolescents were to make changes to their sleep pattern. This approach may elicit the beginning of "change talk."[57,59]

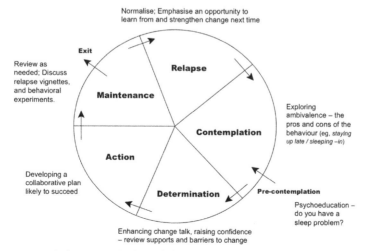

Fig. 9. Stages of motivational change applied to adolescents' sleep behaviors.

Some adolescents will then move to the Determination stage whereby they use more change talk (eg, "I have to change," "I need to make a change," "I can't stay this way"). The clinician is encouraged to praise and reinforce adolescents' change talk[57] and identify ways to support a change in behaviors (eg, enlisting parents or friends), and identify barriers (eg, no access to sufficiently bright light) to increase their confidence that they can change. Care is needed when forming a bright-light therapy or melatonin treatment plan if an adolescent is not completely ready for the Action stage, otherwise the adolescent is unlikely to comply.

The Action and Maintenance stages have already been described above to some extent, in that adolescents act on treatment plans; it is also helpful to inform the adolescent that relapse may occur, but this does not constitute failure. Instead, it is considered a learning opportunity that can elucidate factors contributing to relapse (socializing late with a particular friend, rising too early [ie, before core temperature minimum] with consequent exposure to phase-delaying bright light, and so forth). Revisions of the treatment plan should be developed to anticipate such factors and avoid them during the first weeks of treatment. However, it should be kept in mind that although these motivational techniques may be clinically useful, there is limited evidence for their use in adolescents with sleep problems,[56] and no studies of adolescents with DSPD.

SUMMARY

DSPD is the most common condition with which adolescents present to sleep clinics. Recent innovations in phase-advancing the delayed circadian rhythm include: (1) commercial availability of home assessment of DLMO with sequential salivary melatonin assays, which allows for specific timing of evening melatonin administration based on markers of circadian biology; and (2) bright-light therapy with short-wavelength (green) LED glasses. There is also good evidence to support the use of broad-spectrum white light, as well as sunlight, to phase-advance adolescents' sleep timing. The authors encourage clinicians to be cautious of long-acting melatonin preparations because they may inadvertently worsen the phase delay, and to be wary of chronotherapy because of the limited available evidence. Finally, although more evidence is needed to support its use, motivational interviewing may be a useful technique to supplement the aforementioned treatment strategies.

ACKNOWLEDGMENTS

The authors gratefully thank the adolescents and their families who have participated in past research to help inform current practitioners, who in turn may help future adolescents improve their sleep health.

REFERENCES

1. Crowley SJ, Acebo C, Carskadon MA. Sleep, circadian rhythms, and delayed phase in adolescence. Sleep Med 2007;6:602–12.
2. Lack LC, Wright HR. Clinical management of delayed sleep phase disorder. Behav Sleep Med 2007;5:57–76.
3. Richardson GS, Malin HV. Circadian rhythm sleep disorders: pathophysiology and treatment. J Clin Neurophysiol 1996;13:17–31.
4. Sack RL, Auckley D, Auger RR, et al. Circadian rhythm sleep disorders: part 2, advanced sleep phase disorder, delayed sleep phase disorder, free-running disorder, and irregular sleep-wake rhythm. Sleep 2007;30:1484–501.
5. Wyatt JK. Delayed sleep phase syndrome: pathophysiology and treatment options. Sleep 2004;27:1195–203.
6. Lack LC, Wright HR, Bootzin RR. Delayed sleep-phase disorder. Sleep Med Clin 2009;4:229–39.
7. Bjorvatn B, Pallesen S. A practical approach to circadian rhythm sleep disorders. Sleep Med Rev 2009;13:47–60.
8. Gradisar M, Crowley SJ. Delayed sleep phase disorder in youth. Curr Opin Psychiatry 2013;26:580–5.
9. Weitzman ED, Czeisler CA, Coleman RM, et al. Delayed sleep phase syndrome. A chronobiological disorder with sleep-onset insomnia. Arch Gen Psychiatry 1981;38:737–46.
10. Wilhemsen-Langeland A, Dundas I, Saxvig IW, et al. Psychosocial challenges related to delayed sleep phase disorder. Open Sleep J 2012;5:51–8.
11. Gradisar M, Gardner G, Dohnt H. Recent worldwide sleep patterns and problems during adolescence: a review and meta-analysis of age, region, and sleep. Sleep Med 2011;12:110–8.
12. Carskadon MA. Patterns of sleep and sleepiness in adolescents. Pediatrician 1990;17:5–12.
13. Short MA, Gradisar M, Wright H, et al. Time for bed: parent-set bedtimes associated with improved sleep and daytime functioning in adolescents. Sleep 2011;34:797–800.
14. Crowley SJ, Carskadon MA. Modifications to weekend recovery sleep delay circadian phase in older adolescents. Chronobiol Int 2010;27:1469–92.
15. Taylor DJ, Jenni OG, Acebo C, et al. Sleep tendency during extended wakefulness: insights into

adolescent sleep regulation and behaviour. J Sleep Res 2005;14:239–44.

16. American Psychiatric Association. Diagnostic and statistical manual of mental disorders. 5th edition. Arlington, VA: American Psychiatric Association; 2013.

17. American Academy of Sleep Medicine. The international classification of sleep disorders, 2nd edition: diagnostic and coding manual. Westchester (IL): American Academy of Sleep Medicine; 2005.

18. Acebo C, Sadeh A, Seifer R, et al. Estimating sleep patterns with activity monitoring in children and adolescents: how many nights are necessary for reliable measures? Sleep 1999;22:95–103.

19. Sadeh A, Sharkey KM, Carskadon MA. Activity-based sleep-wake identification: an empirical test of methodological issues. Sleep 1994;17:201–7.

20. Ancoli-Israel S, Cole R, Alessi C, et al. The role of actigraphy in the study of sleep and circadian rhythms. Sleep 2003;26:342–92.

21. Short MA, Gradisar M, Lack LC, et al. The discrepancy between actigraphic and sleep diary measures of sleep in adolescents. Sleep Med 2012; 13:378–84.

22. Saxvig IW, Wilhelmsen-Langeland A, Pallesen S, et al. Objective measures of sleep and dim light melatonin onset in adolescents and young adults with delayed sleep phase disorder compared to healthy controls. J Sleep Res 2013;22:365–72.

23. Lewy AJ, Wehr TA, Goodwin FK, et al. Light suppresses melatonin secretion in humans. Science 1980;210:1267–9.

24. Lewy AJ, Sack RL, Blood ML, et al. Melatonin marks circadian phase position and resets the endogenous circadian pacemaker in humans. Ciba Found Symp 1995;183:303–17.

25. Lewy AJ, Cutler NL, Sack RL. The endogenous melatonin profile as a marker for circadian phase position. J Biol Rhythms 1999;14:227–36.

26. Keijzer H, Smits MG, Peeters T, et al. Evaluation of salivary melatonin measurements for dim light melatonin onset calculations in patients with possible sleep-wake rhythm disorders. Clin Chim Acta 2011;412:1616–20.

27. Pullman RE, Roepke SE, Duffy JF. Laboratory validation of an in-home method for assessing circadian phase using dim light melatonin onset (DLMO). Sleep Med 2012;13:703–6.

28. Reiter RJ, Tan DX. What constitutes a physiological concentration of melatonin? J Pineal Res 2003;34: 79–80.

29. Nagtegaal E, Peeters T, Swart W, et al. Correlation between concentrations of melatonin in saliva and serum in patients with delayed sleep phase syndrome. Ther Drug Monit 1998;20:181.

30. Benloucif S, Guico MJ, Reid KJ, et al. Stability of melatonin and temperature as circadian phase

markers and their relation to sleep times in humans. J Biol Rhythms 2005;20:178–88.

31. Gradisar M, Dohnt H, Gardner G, et al. A randomized controlled trial of cognitive-behavior therapy plus bright light therapy for adolescent delayed sleep phase disorder. Sleep 2011;34:1671–80.

32. Johns M. A new method for measuring daytime sleepiness: the Epworth Sleepiness Scale. Sleep 1991;14:540–5.

33. Wilhelmsen-Langeland A, Saxvig IW, Pallesen S, et al. A randomized controlled trial with bright light and melatonin for the treatment of delayed sleep phase disorder: effects on subjective and objective sleepiness and cognitive function. J Biol Rhythms 2013;28:306–21.

34. Drake C, Nickel C, Burduvali E, et al. The Pediatric Sleepiness Scale (PDSS): sleep habits and school outcomes in middle-school children. Sleep 2003; 26:455–8.

35. Short MA, Gradisar M, Lack LC, et al. The sleep patterns and well-being of Australian adolescents. J Adolesc 2013;36:103–10.

36. Meijer AM. Chronic sleep reduction, functioning at school and school achievement in preadolescents. J Sleep Res 2008;17:395–405.

37. Dewald JF, Short MA, Gradisar M, et al. The Chronic Sleep Reduction Questionnaire (CSRQ): a cross-cultural comparison and validation in Dutch and Australian adolescents. J Sleep Res 2012;21:584–94.

38. van Maanen A, Dewald-Kaufmann JF, Smits MG, et al. Chronic sleep reduction in adolescents with delayed sleep phase disorder and effects of melatonin treatment. Sleep Biol Rhythms 2013;11: 99–104.

39. Saxvig IW, Wilhelmsen-Langeland A, Pallesen S, et al. A randomized controlled trial with bright light and melatonin for delayed sleep phase disorder: effects on subjective and objective sleep. Chronobiol Int 2014;31:72–86.

40. Heath M, Sutherland C, Bartel K, et al. Does one hour of bright or short-wavelength filtered tablet screenlight have a meaningful effect on adolescents' prebedtime alertness, sleep and daytime functioning? Chronobiol Int 2014;31(4):496–505.

41. Wood B, Rea MS, Plitnick B, et al. Light level and duration of exposure determine the impact of self-luminous tablets on melatonin suppression. Appl Ergon 2013;44:237–40.

42. Wright HR, Lack LC, Kennaway DJ. Differential effects of light wavelength in phase advancing the melatonin rhythm. J Pineal Res 2003;36:140–4.

43. Burgess HJ, Revell VL, Eastman CI. A three pulse phase response curve to three milligrams of melatonin in humans. J Physiol 2008;586:639–47.

44. Lewy AJ, Ahmed S, Jackson JM, et al. Melatonin shifts human circadian rhythms according to a

phase-response curve. Chronobiol Int 1992;9: 380–92.

45. Mundey K, Benloucif S, Harsanyi K, et al. Phase-dependent treatment of delayed sleep phase syndrome with melatonin. Sleep 2005;28:1271–8.

46. Nagtegaal JE, Kerkhof GA, Smits MG, et al. Delayed sleep phase syndrome: a placebo-controlled cross-over study on the effects of melatonin administered five hours before the individual dim light melatonin onset. J Sleep Res 1998;7:135–43.

47. Braam W, Smits MG, Didden R, et al. Exogenous melatonin for sleep problems in individuals with intellectual disability: a meta-analysis. Dev Med Child Neurol 2009;51:340–9.

48. van Geijlswijk IM, Korzilius HP, Smits MG. The use of exogenous melatonin in delayed sleep phase disorder: a meta-analysis. Sleep 2010;33:1605–14.

49. Buscemi N, Vandermeer B, Hooton N, et al. Efficacy and safety of exogenous melatonin for secondary sleep disorders and sleep disorders accompanying sleep restriction: meta-analysis. BMJ 2006;332:385–93.

50. Lewy AJ. Melatonin as a marker and phase-resetter of circadian rhythms in humans. Adv Exp Med Biol 2002;460:425–34.

51. Keijzer H, Smits MG, Duffy JF, et al. Why the dim light melatonin onset (DLMO) should be measured before treatment of patients with circadian rhythm sleep disorders. Sleep Med Rev 2013. http://dx.doi.org/10.1016/j.smrv.2013.12.001.

52. Neurim Pharmaceuticals. Prescribing information. 2013. Available at: http://www.ema.europa.eu/docs/en_GB/document_library/EPAR_-_Product_Information/human/000695/WC500026811.pdf. Accessed March 12, 2014.

53. Czeisler CA, Richardson GS, Coleman RM, et al. Chronotherapy: resetting the circadian clocks of patients with delayed sleep phase insomnia. Sleep 1981;4:1–21.

54. Short MA, Gradisar M, Gill J, et al. Identifying adolescent sleep problems. PLoS One 2013;8: e75301.

55. Bootzin RR, Stevens SJ. Adolescents, substance abuse, and the treatment of insomnia and daytime sleepiness. Clin Psychol Rev 2005;25:629–44.

56. Cain N, Gradisar M, Moseley L. A motivational school-based sleep intervention of adolescent sleep problems. Sleep Med 2011;12:246–51.

57. Miller WR, Rollnick S. Motivational interviewing: preparing people for change. 2nd edition. New York: Guilford Press; 2002.

58. Dewald JF, Meijer AM, Oort FJ, et al. The influence of sleep quality, sleep duration and sleepiness on school performance in children and adolescents: a meta-analytic review. Sleep Med 2010;14: 179–89.

59. Amrhein PC, Miller WR, Yahne CE, et al. Client commitment language during motivational interviewing predicts drug use outcomes. J Consult Clin Psychol 2003;71:862–78.

Quality of Life in Children with Narcolepsy and Cataplexy

Michel Lecendreux, MD[a,b,*]

KEYWORDS

- Sleep • Narcolepsy • Child • Quality of life • Cataplexy

KEY POINTS

- Narcolepsy is a chronic and disabling neurologic disorder that affects sleep and wakefulness and is characterized by excessive daytime sleepiness (EDS), sudden sleep episodes, and attacks of muscle atonia mostly triggered by emotions (cataplexy).
- Narcolepsy is a lifelong nonprogressive disorder, the onset of which occurs not infrequently during childhood. However, narcolepsy in children is frequently underdiagnosed or misdiagnosed.
- Since a signal regarding the potential association between H1N1 vaccination and narcolepsy was raised in Sweden and Finland, additional cases have been reported in different countries across Europe and particularly in France.
- Young patients affected by the disorder often show dramatic and abrupt impairment in their social skills and academic performance because of excessive daytime sleepiness, fatigue, and lack of energy.
- Underrecognition and undertreatment of narcolepsy represents a significant unmet medical need in childhood.

INTRODUCTION

As in adults, pediatric narcolepsy may show a great deal of variability in its presentation. Symptoms may start abruptly and sometimes dramatically with the sudden occurrence of extreme sleepiness and complete cataplexy, or progressively and insidiously, with excessive daytime sleepiness (EDS) or weight gain being the only symptoms over weeks or months. Although cataplexy is the most specific symptom of the disorder, it is usually not the first symptom to appear and may not be manifested for some 1 to 5 years after EDS occurs. This variability in presentation often leads to difficulties in recognizing the condition or making the diagnosis at an early stage.

Narcolepsy in children, therefore, is frequently underdiagnosed or mistaken for other diseases, and may not even be considered in the differential diagnosis of the presenting complaint.[1] Young patients affected by the disorder often show dramatic and abrupt impairments in many domains because of EDS, fatigue, and lack of energy, including social skills and academic performance.[2] This situation thus represents a significant unmet medical need in childhood.

PREVALENCE OF PEDIATRIC NARCOLEPSY

The incidence of narcolepsy in adults (<1 per 100,000 new cases per year) suggests that it is a rare condition; however, given that it is also a

Disclosure Statement: Dr M. Lecendreux has received funds for speaking and board engagements with UCB Pharma, Jazz, and Bioprojet.
a Pediatric Sleep Center, Hospital Robert Debré, Paris, France; b National Reference Centre for Orphan Diseases, Narcolepsy, Idiopathic Hypersomnia and Kleine-Levin Syndrome (CNR Narcolepsie-Hypersomnie), France
* Pediatric Sleep Center, Hospital Robert Debré, Paris, France.
E-mail address: michel.lecendreux@rdb.aphp.fr

Sleep Med Clin 9 (2014) 211–217
http://dx.doi.org/10.1016/j.jsmc.2014.03.001

chronic disorder, the prevalence is much greater at 20 to 60 per 100,000 in Western countries. The prevalence of the disorder in children remains unknown. Based on a study conducted in the United States, the disorder could affect some 20 to 50 per 100,000 children.[3] Although narcolepsy has traditionally been considered to be a disease of adulthood, most cases have their onset in childhood or adolescence.[4,5]

Recently, systematic approaches have been established to study narcolepsy in childhood and adolescence. A French national database was created in 2007 (research program Narcobank, French Grant PHRC AOM07-138 from the French Health Ministry, Assistance Publique-Hôpitaux de Paris) that has thus far gathered clinical data on more than 100 children and adolescents aged 5 to 16 years with narcolepsy. The cohort was composed of 117 children (65 boys) with a mean age of 11.6 ± 3.1 years at time of diagnosis. The gender ratio was 0.56 in favor of males versus females. The children were followed up in different French expert orphan disease sleep centers for narcolepsy management, including the Robert Debré Children's Hospital in Paris, the Mother-Children's Hospital in Lyon, the Gui-de-Chauliac Adult's Hospital in Montpellier, and the Pitié-Salpétrière Adult's Hospital in Paris. The considerable number of patients enrolled in this database demonstrates that narcolepsy is far from exceptional in children and adolescents and should always be suspected when a youngster presents with abnormal daytime sleepiness or partial or complete loss of muscle tone triggered by emotions.

Primary care pediatricians can play a significant role in the care of patients with narcolepsy in regards to appropriate diagnosis and optimal management. Available treatments have been shown to be effective in clinical settings; however, lack of treatment can result in an increased risk of poor outcomes. For example, the tendency for increased weight gain is intrinsic to childhood narcolepsy and is manifested relatively early in the course of the disorder. Early identification and management of weight gain could thus prevent such significant consequences as morbid obesity[6] and even potentially precocious puberty.[7]

DEMOGRAPHICS OF CHILDHOOD NARCOLEPSY

Narcolepsy in children has been reported in a wide variety of ethnic groups, including white Americans and Europeans, Japanese, Korean, Mexican, and Chinese populations. For example, recent narcolepsy-cataplexy (NC) case studies have included reports on disease characteristics in both white children and Chinese children younger than 13 years of age.[8] Another study reported on the presentation of cataplexy in 23 young Italian patients.[9] Although this finding should be interpreted in light of recent immigration rates, in our own database we found a high proportion of patients (representing some 26% of the cohort) originating from Sub-Saharan Africa, especially Mali, Cameroon, or Benin. White patients represented 33% of our cohort, with the remaining originating from the French Indies (24%), North African Maghreb countries (10%), and Comoro Islands (3%).

NARCOLEPSY AND AGE OF ONSET

Early observations in the United States[10] and Japan[11] reported that approximately 50% of patients with narcolepsy had an onset before 15 years of age, with less than 10% with an onset before 5 years of age. Similarly, in a database of 1219 cases reported by Aran and colleagues,[12] although less than 10% were children (<18 years) at evaluation, 40% reported an onset before 15 years of age and 2.1% had an onset before 5 years of age (1.1% with cataplexy onset before age 5 years). In our own database of 117 children and adolescents affected by narcolepsy with or without cataplexy, the age range was 5.4 to 16.6 years and the mean age at disease onset was 9.2 years (±6.2).

Although the occurrence of narcolepsy has been reported in children during the first year of life, very early onset cases are anecdotal and most often secondary to comorbid brain disorders, including tumors or abnormalities localized most frequently to the diencephalon or to the brainstem. Niemann-Pick disease type C is often associated with early onset cataplexy.[13] Another cause of very early onset of secondary cataplexy is craniopharyngioma, which accounts for 9% of all pediatric intracranial tumors overall.

Importantly, it seems that the delay between the onset of narcolepsy symptoms and diagnosis is lower in childhood than in adulthood. Early adult studies in the 1980s to 1990s reported a median delay between onset of symptoms and diagnosis of more than 10 years[14]; a similar delay was also reported in the French Harmony study.[15] However, in the Narcobank cohort, we found a mean duration of symptoms before diagnosis of 31 months, and in three children the diagnosis had been made within 5 months after the first occurrence of narcoleptic symptoms (ie, abrupt cataplexy or sleep attack but excluding possible weight gain).

This is potentially very important because children diagnosed shortly after symptom onset may be preferential candidates for immunotherapy based on high-dose intravenous immuno-globulin administration, as has been previously recommended.[16,17]

NARCOLEPSY AND THE IMPACT OF H1N1 VACCINATION AND INFECTION

In August 2010, the Medicinal Product Authority in Sweden announced a special investigation regarding the onset of narcolepsy after H1N1 vaccine. During the summer of 2010, the Medicinal Product Authority received a total of 22 reports of narcolepsy as an adverse reaction after influenza (A) H1N1 Pandemrix vaccination.[18,19] The reports included children aged 12 to 16 years in whom symptoms compatible with narcolepsy, diagnosed after thorough medical investigation, occurred 1 to 2 months after vaccination.

Clinical features were mostly identical in post- and non–post-H1N1 vaccinated children. The onset of symptoms (EDS) was accurately reported by parents in most cases, and these symptoms were often preceded by an uncharacteristic weight gain and followed by the occurrence of cataplexy triggered by emotion a few weeks or months later. Hypotonia of the face and the jaw (persistent hypotonia with complex movement disorder) was also reported in many of the children. Other potential triggering factors were excluded by thorough history taking and all patients had normal brain magnetic resonance imaging scans. Furthermore, all of the pediatric patients who had HLA DQB1*0602 testing and cerebrospinal hypocretin levels had positive antigen levels and were deficient in hypocretin. Gender or Tanner staging did not seem to have any influence.[20]

Similar cases have also been reported in many European countries. In Finland, for example, more than 100 new cases, mostly children showing typical NC features, have so far been reported after exposure to H1N1 vaccination.[21] As a result of these studies, the incidence of the disease was estimated to be more than 4 per 100,000 after the H1N1 vaccination campaign, compared with previous estimates of 0.3 per 100,000; the estimated risk for developing narcolepsy after Pandemrix vaccination was 1 per 4000.

In France, using a dynamic retrospective case-control cohort study, we reported a strong association between Pandemrix adjuvanted AS03 H1N1 vaccine and narcolepsy with cataplexy in children and in adults. Our results showed that H1N1 vaccination, mostly Pandemrix adjuvanted AS03 vaccine, contributed to NC in children and adults; but with only 28 cases reported at that time, there were potential associations with other environmental factors in genetically predisposed subjects with HLA DQB1*0602.[22]

In a recent Chinese narcolepsy cohort consisting of 906 well-characterized patients, most of whom were diagnosed as children,[23] the onset of narcolepsy seemed to occur at an early age, and the development of symptoms was frequently abrupt. It was also found that the occurrence of narcolepsy onset was three to four times greater than predicted following the 2009 to 2010 winter season, when the H1N1 pandemic was at its peak. Most new narcolepsy patients in 2010 (96%) did not report a prior H1N1 vaccination. Most of these cases were young children.

In November of 2013, a new European Alliance was formed on behalf of those children and adults who have developed narcolepsy or other debilitating illnesses as a result of the human H1N1 vaccine (Pandemrix). Recommendations arising from the conference included promotion of individual government and industry support and adequate financial compensation for victims to restore their quality of life (QOL) and to allow them to reach their full potential.

PEDIATRIC NARCOLEPSY AND QOL

Narcolepsy in adults is known to be associated with a high socioeconomic burden comparable with other chronic neurologic diseases, with indirect costs being considerably higher than direct costs.[24] However, the exact health care financial burden caused by pediatric narcolepsy is not known. Moreover, accurate determination of health care costs is confounded by the problem of lack of timely recognition and accurate diagnosis of narcolepsy. Thus, costs might be overestimated if children are diagnosed inappropriately and receive treatment that may not benefit them; however, costs might be underestimated if significant a proportion of children go undiagnosed.

In the adult population, the health and social consequences of narcolepsy have been evaluated in several studies; these suggest that the accumulation of clinical symptoms and the "social dysfunction" associated with the disease could result in a deterioration in physical and psychosocial function and emotional health in these patients, and thus have considerable impact on QOL.[15,25–28]

Only a few studies have focused on pediatric narcolepsy and QOL. Stores and colleagues[29] studied the impact of narcolepsy on health-related QOL (HRQL) in children. As a multidimensional measure, HRQL attempts to identify the most relevant aspects of health, which in adolescence are physical and emotional well-being and self-esteem, and social functioning perception with peers, parents, and teachers. The psychosocial impact of narcolepsy and difficulty in coping with sleepiness could also expose patients to the risk of exogenous depression. Behavioral problems, emotional problems with depression, and social difficulties have been reported in 33%, 44%, and 66%, respectively, of narcoleptic children in different series.[12,30,31]

In a recent study performed by our group,[32] HRQL was assessed using a questionnaire adapted for adolescents (Vécu et Santé Perçue de l'Adolescent [VSP-A]),[33] for children (VSP-E), and for parents (VSP-P).[34] VSP-A[2,25] is a self-report questionnaire for adolescents aged 11 to 18 years that includes several domains including psychological and physical well-being, body image, vitality, relationships (friends, parents, teachers, medical staff), leisure, school performance, and a global HRQL index. Lower scores correspond to a poorer QOL. VSP-P can also be filled out by parents.[35] The VSP-A was adapted for children (8–10 years; VSP-E)[36] with the domains of general well-being, energy, self-image, relationships, leisure, school, and global HRQL index. This corresponds to the HRQL index of adolescents minus romantic relationships and relations with teachers. These questionnaires were validated in 1057 healthy adolescents without acute or chronic diseases (mean age, 14.8 years; gender ratio, 0.9) and 663 healthy children (mean age, 10.3 years; gender ratio, 0.9) in the French population.[34]

In our study, 53 narcoleptic adolescents, 31 children, and 83 parents filled out these questionnaires. The characteristics of this subsample were comparable with those of the French population attending school in regards to age, gender, grade, and socioeconomic status.[33] Results show that narcolepsy impacts HRQL across several domains, especially in children. The narcoleptic patients reported lower HRQL on VSP-A scores than healthy control subjects on vitality and physical well-being, and on the general HRQL index. Narcoleptic patients, especially younger patients, reported fewer leisure activities compared with healthy subjects, not surprising given their lower scores on physical well-being and vitality. These results are consistent with those reported in the literature comparing healthy with ill pediatric patients.[37,38]

In addition, girls with narcolepsy were found to have lower scores than boys. Compared with children, adolescents with narcolepsy had higher scores for the dimensions dealing with relations with friends and lower scores on school performance. However, compared with the general population, the differences between children and adolescents were relatively minor, likely caused by the lower overall HRQL of youth with narcolepsy.

We also found that cataplexy did not show any correlation with HRQL scales,[25,38,39] although it should be noted that there were few patients with narcolepsy without cataplexy in our sample. This finding corroborates the similarity in HRQL profiles in pediatric narcolepsy reported by Stores and colleagues.[29] Disease duration, delay in diagnosis, therapy status (taking drugs for narcolepsy or not), and obesity did not reach any statistically significant correlation with HRQL.

NONPHARMACOLOGIC INTERVENTIONS FOR PEDIATRIC NARCOLEPSY

Although pharmacologic treatments targeting EDS, cataplexy, and fragmented nocturnal sleep are well-studied in and mainstays of treatment of adults with narcolepsy, none of these medications are indicated for use in children. Thus, although extensive "off-label" use does exist in pediatric clinical practice, it is especially important to include nonphamacologic strategies in the management of children and adolescents.

Scheduled Naps

Although no studies demonstrating their effectiveness are available, measures aimed at enabling one or more daytime sleep periods are generally recommended. One to two scheduled naps of 20 to 30 minutes increase daytime wakefulness and improve psychomotor performance. Clinical experience suggests that most children and adolescents benefit from at least one brief scheduled daytime nap during school. Naps are often scheduled immediately after lunch, and should take place in a quiet dedicated room where the child is able to lie down and rest on a bed (ie, not in the classroom). The child should be supervised during each nap and awakened by a responsible adult (teacher, school nurse) after 20 to 30 minutes, depending on the age of the child and the severity of the symptoms. It is important to ensure that late afternoon naps (after school) do not interfere with nighttime sleep periods.

Sleep Practices

Encouragement of healthy sleep practices is a key component of the daily management of all pediatric patients with narcolepsy. These include the following:

- Schedule a sufficient "window" for sleep (bedtime and wake time) to meet sleep needs
- Keep consistent bedtimes and wake times on school and nonschool days
- Maintain a regular schedule of daytime activities
- Have a regular bedtime routine
- Avoid light exposure in the evening before bedtime, including electronics
- Increase light exposure in the morning on waking

Nutrition and Exercise

Weight gain and obesity are frequently observed in children with narcolepsy, with cataplexy at disease onset, especially in younger patients. Obesity in turn may impact negatively on sleep efficiency and is associated with increased school absenteeism. Obese children also have a higher risk of sleep-disordered breathing. Thus, prevention and treatment of weight problems in these children are imperative, and include careful monitoring of weight gain. Nutritional recommendations and healthy eating strategies, including regular mealtimes, should be provided to the child and the family on an ongoing basis by a nutritionist or dietician to avoid weight gain and to help maintain regular growth.

Adequate physical activity should also be encouraged in pediatric patients with narcolepsy to reduce the risk of weight gain and build muscle strength. However, patients with poorly controlled cataplexy may require extra supervision and may need to refrain from potentially unsafe physical activities until their symptoms are better managed. Physiotherapy may also be helpful, especially in addressing posture when sitting in the classroom.

Psychological Interventions

Counseling, including family therapy or brief psychotherapy, is often helpful in enabling the child and family to accept the loss of their previous healthy state and progressively accept the reality of a disabling chronic condition. Specific techniques based on cognitive behavior therapy may be helpful in developing coping strategies, such as assisting the child in identifying and anticipating specific triggers for cataplectic attacks (eg, laughter, surprise, anger). Family and/or individual therapy may be particularly useful in addressing challenges during the transition in adolescence to greater independence (driving, sexual activity, medication adherence, and so forth). Group therapy has also been proposed to encourage modeling in children or adolescents presenting with chronic diseases; these groups often focus on coping strategies, adherence to treatment, and social interactions. Patient support organizations, such as the Narcolepsy Network and Wake Up Narcolepsy, often sponsor local support group meetings; these allow patients and families to share information and encourage young patients to exchange advice and ideas on managing their disease and to interact with peers. Internet forums, specialty camps, and regional or national meetings are other vehicles often sponsored by patient advocacy organizations that can play a crucial role in helping patients and families. The following is adapted for pediatric narcolepsy patients from The Incredible Years teacher classroom management (TCM) program:

Recommendations in the classroom and home settings to improve QOL

1. Strengthen social skills and appropriate play skills (encourage leisure activities, such as sports, artistic activities, dynamic group interactions).

2. Provide a classroom atmosphere whenever possible in which the child is less likely to fall asleep. Engage the child in activities that encourage him or her to be engaged and involved instead of sleepy and bored.

3. Promote the child's use of self-control strategies, such as effective problem-solving and anger or frustration management.

4. Children with narcolepsy are often teased by peers for falling asleep or having cataplectic attacks. Model adaptive ways to interact with peers under these negative circumstances.

5. Increase emotional awareness by labeling feelings and promoting recognition of differing perspectives. Help the child to recognize signs of sleepiness and fatigue in themselves and others.

6. Boost the likelihood of school readiness and academic success by increasing alertness and/or encouraging assistance from family members and peers when appropriate to prevent involuntary dozing off during the day or to help the child to focus on a specific task.

7. Discourage and deflect acting-out behaviors (aggression, noncompliance) as a means of expressing frustration.

8. Address the child's negative cognitive attributions and conflict management approaches (ie, encourage the child to think positively about their disease and to seek out support from parents and teachers, and from classmates and friends when appropriate).

9. Increase self-esteem and self-confidence. Increased resilience offers protection from various mental health symptoms, such as depression and anxiety. Resilience can also help offset factors that increase the risk of mental health conditions, such as lack of social support, being bullied, or previous trauma.

SUMMARY AND DIRECTIONS FOR FUTURE RESEARCH

Narcolepsy is not rare in children and adolescents and is a disabling and lifelong disorder that may significantly impact the QOL of these children from a very young age. A healthy lifestyle and regular waking and sleep routines are strongly recommended for children and adolescents suffering from narcolepsy. Nonpharmacologic interventions should be systematically evaluated as treatment approaches. The ultimate aim of these endeavors should be to improve the outlook and prognosis for children and adolescents suffering from narcolepsy with or without cataplexy.

Future research should focus on effective behavioral and cognitive therapies for sleep disruption and deficits in alertness in children with narcolepsy. Novel strategies for helping children to adapt to and manage their disease are needed. At the present time only a handful of the sleep centers and/or neurology practices managing these children are able to provide dedicated psychological help for children and adolescents suffering from narcolepsy. Evidence-based guidelines should be developed for health professionals, parents, teachers, and patients.

REFERENCES

1. Guilleminault C, Pelayo R. Narcolepsy in prepubertal children. Ann Neurol 1998;43:135–42 [PubMed ID: 9450782].
2. Hayes D Jr. Narcolepsy with cataplexy in early childhood. Clin Pediatr (Phila) 2006;45:361–3 [PubMed ID: 16703160].
3. Silber MH, Krahn LE, Olson EJ, et al. The epidemiology of narcolepsy in Olmsted County, Minnesota: a population-based study. Sleep 2002;25:197–202 [PubMed ID: 11902429].
4. Young D, Zorick F, Wittig R, et al. Narcolepsy in a pediatric population. Am J Dis Child 1988;142:210–3 [PubMed ID: 3341326].
5. Challamel MJ, Mazzola ME, Nevsimalova S, et al. Narcolepsy in children. Sleep 1994;17:S17–20 [PubMed ID: 7701194].
6. Perriol MP, Cartigny M, Lamblin MD, et al. Childhood-onset narcolepsy, obesity and puberty in four consecutive children: a close temporal link. J Pediatr Endocrinol Metab 2010;23:257–65 [PubMed ID: 20480724].
7. Plazzi G, Parmeggiani A, Mignot E, et al. Narcolepsy-cataplexy associated with precocious puberty. Neurology 2006;66:1577–9 [PubMed ID: 16717224].
8. Han F, Lin L, Li J, et al. Presentations of primary hypersomnia in Chinese children. Sleep 2011;34:627–32 [PubMed ID: 21532956].
9. Serra L, Montagna P, Mignot E, et al. Cataplexy features in childhood narcolepsy. Mov Disord 2008;23:858–65 [PubMed ID: 18307264].
10. Yoss RE, Daly DD. Narcolepsy in children. Pediatrics 1960;25:1025–33 [PubMed ID: 13846589].
11. Honda Y, Asaka A, Tanimura M, et al. A genetic study of narcolepsy and excessive daytime sleepiness in 308 families with a narcolepsy or hypersomnia proband. In: Guilleminault C, Lugaresi E, editors. Sleep/wake disorders: natural history, epidemiology and long-term evolution. New York: Raven Press; 1983. p. 187–99.
12. Aran A, Einen M, Lin L, et al. Clinical and therapeutic aspects of childhood narcolepsy-cataplexy: a retrospective study of 51 children. Sleep 2010;33(11):1457–64 [PubMed ID: 21102987].
13. Smit LS, Lammers GJ, Catsman-Berrevoets CE. Cataplexy leading to the diagnosis of Niemann-Pick disease type C. Pediatr Neurol 2006;35:82–4 [PubMed ID: 16814094].
14. Morrish E, King MA, Smith IE, et al. Factors associated with a delay in the diagnosis of narcolepsy. Sleep Med 2004;5:37–41 [PubMed ID: 14725825].
15. Dauvilliers Y, Paquereau J, Bastuji H, et al. Psychological health in central hypersomnias: the French Harmony study. J Neurol Neurosurg Psychiatry 2009;80:636–41 [PubMed ID: 19211597].
16. Dauvilliers Y, Carlander B, Rivier F, et al. Successful management of cataplexy with intravenous immunoglobulins at narcolepsy onset. Ann Neurol 2004;56:905–8 [PubMed ID: 15562415].
17. Lecendreux M, Maret S, Bassetti C, et al. Clinical efficacy of high-dose intravenous immunoglobulins near the onset of narcolepsy in a 10-year-old boy. J Sleep Res 2003;12:347–8 [PubMed ID: 14633248].
18. Bardage C, Persson I, Ortqvist A, et al. Neurological and autoimmune disorders after vaccination against pandemic influenza A (H1N1) with a monovalent adjuvanted vaccine: population based cohort study in Stockholm, Sweden. BMJ 2011;343:d5956 [PubMed ID: 21994316].
19. Montastruc JL, Durrieu G, Rascol O. Pandemrix°, (H1N1)v influenza and reported cases of narcolepsy. Vaccine 2011;29:2010 [PubMed ID: 21232649].
20. Lecendreux M, Franco P, Arnulf I, et al. Possible relation between (A) H1N1 vaccination and pediatric narcolepsy [Abstract 0820]. Sleep 2011;34(Abstract Supplement):A281.
21. Tsai TF, Crucitti A, Nacci P, et al. Explorations of clinical trials and pharmacovigilance databases of MF59(R)-adjuvanted influenza vaccines for associated cases of narcolepsy. Scand J Infect Dis 2011;43:702–6 [PubMed ID: 21534891].
22. Dauvilliers Y, Arnulf I, Lecendreux M, et al, Narcoflu-VF study group. Increased risk of narcolepsy in children and adults after pandemic H1N1 vaccination in

France. Brain 2013;136(Pt 8):2486–96. http://dx.doi.org/10.1093/brain/awt187 [PubMedID: 23884811].

23. Han F, Lin L, Warby SC, et al. Narcolepsy onset is seasonal and increased following the 2009 H1N1 pandemic in China. Ann Neurol 2011;70:410–7 [PubMed ID: 21866560].

24. Dodel R, Peter H, Walbert T, et al. The socioeconomic impact of narcolepsy. Sleep 2004;27:1123–8 [PubMed ID: 15532206].

25. Daniels E, King MA, Smith IE, et al. Health-related quality of life in narcolepsy. J Sleep Res 2001; 10(1):75–81.

26. Vignatelli L, D'Alessandro R, Mosconi P, et al. Health-related quality of life in Italian patients with narcolepsy: the SF-36 health survey. Sleep Med 2004;5(5):467–75.

27. Vignatelli L, Plazzi G, Peschechera F, et al. A 5-year prospective cohort study on health-related quality of life in patients with narcolepsy. Sleep Med 2011; 12(1):19–23.

28. Dodel R, Peter H, Spottke A, et al. Health-related quality of life in patients with narcolepsy. Sleep Med 2007;8(7–8):733–41.

29. Stores G, Montgomery P, Wiggs L. The psychosocial problems of children with narcolepsy and those with excessive daytime sleepiness of uncertain origin. Pediatrics 2006;118(4):e1116–23.

30. Nevsimalova S, Jara C, Prihodova I, et al. Clinical features of childhood narcolepsy. Can cataplexy be foretold? Eur J Paediatr Neurol 2011;15(4):320–5.

31. Peraita-Adrados R, Garcia-Penas J, Ruiz-Falco L, et al. Clinical, polysomnographic and laboratory characteristics of narcolepsy-cataplexy in a sample of children and adolescents. Sleep Med 2011;12(1): 24–7.

32. Inocente C, Gustin MP, Lavault S, et al. Quality of life in children with narcolepsy. CNS Neurosci Ther, in press.

33. Simeoni MC, Auquier P, Antoniotti S, et al. Validation of a French health-related quality of life instrument for adolescents: the VSP-A. Qual Life Res 2000; 9(4):393–403.

34. Gras D. Santé et qualité de vie des frères et soeurs d'enfants atteints de maladies chroniques. Nantes: 2009.

35. Simeoni MC, Sapin C, Antoniotti S, et al. Health-related quality of life reported by French adolescents: a predictive approach of health status? J Adolesc Health 2001;28(4):288–94.

36. Serra-Sutton V, Ferrer M, Rajmil L, et al. Population norms and cut-off-points for suboptimal health related quality of life in two generic measures for adolescents: the Spanish VSP-A and KINDL-R. Health Qual Life Outcomes 2009;7:35.

37. Starfield B, Riley AW, Green BF, et al. The adolescent child health and illness profile. A population-based measure of health. Med Care 1995;33(5): 553–66.

38. Ravens-Sieberer U, Bullinger M. Assessing health-related quality of life in chronically ill children with the German KINDL: first psychometric and content analytical results. Qual Life Res 1998;7(5):399–407.

39. Reinke W, Herman KC, Newcomer L. The Incredible Years Teacher classroom management training: the methods and principle that support fidelity of training delivery. Sch Psychol Rev 2011;40(4): 509–29.

Improving Positive Airway Pressure Adherence in Children

Michelle S. King, MD, Melissa S. Xanthopoulos, PhD,
Carole L. Marcus, MBBCh*

KEYWORDS

- Adherence • Continuous positive airway pressure • Obstructive sleep apnea syndrome • Children
- Behavioral intervention

KEY POINTS

- Obstructive sleep apnea syndrome (OSAS) is a relatively common disorder affecting approximately 1% to 5% of children aged 5 to 13 years, and is associated with adverse neurobehavioral, cognitive, and physiologic consequences.
- Adenotonsillectomy is considered to be the first-line treatment; however, not all patients are surgical candidates and some patients will continue to have symptoms after surgery.
- Continuous positive airway pressure (CPAP) is a safe and effective treatment for children with OSAS who do not improve with surgery or who are not candidates for surgery. The major limiting factor for successful treatment with CPAP is adherence.
- Psychosocial factors and patient characteristics are the main predictors of poor adherence, with low maternal education being the strongest.
- Managing suboptimal adherence entails engaging and educating the child and parent about CPAP; this involves discussing preexisting attitudes, outcome expectations, and side effects, in addition to providing constant support from a dedicated team.
- More intensive cognitive behavioral interventions may prove useful in overcoming poor CPAP adherence in complex cases.

INTRODUCTION

Obstructive sleep apnea syndrome (OSAS) is estimated to affect approximately 1% to 5% of children between the ages of 5 and 13 years.[1–4] OSAS has been shown to contribute to neurobehavioral and cognitive morbidity in children, including poor school performance, impaired language skills, inattention, hyperactivity, and reduced quality of life.[5–10] OSAS is also associated with significant physiologic consequences, including insulin resistance, elevated markers of inflammation, systemic hypertension, and, in severe cases, left ventricular dysfunction and cor pulmonale.[11–17]

Pathophysiologic mechanisms for the development of OSAS can be broadly divided into anatomic factors that reduce the caliber of the upper airway, such as craniofacial abnormalities, obesity, and adenotonsillar hypertrophy, and factors that increase upper-airway collapsibility, such as neurologically based alterations in upper airway muscle tone.[18–20] Deficits in central control of ventilation (eg, Chiari malformation) may also play an etiologic role in some cases.

Disclosures: C.L. Marcus has received funding from Philips Respironics and Ventus, and was funded, in part, by NIH RO1 HL58585. NIHMS-ID: 571573.
Sleep Center, The Children's Hospital of Philadelphia, Perelman School of Medicine, University of Pennsylvania, 34th and Civic Center Boulevard, Philadelphia, PA 19104, USA
* Corresponding author.
E-mail address: MARCUS@email.chop.edu

INDICATIONS FOR POSITIVE AIRWAY PRESSURE

The primary risk factors for OSAS in children are distinct from those in the adult population, with adenotonsillar hypertrophy being implicated in most childhood cases.[21–23] Adenotonsillectomy is therefore considered to be the first-line treatment for otherwise healthy children with OSAS.[1] A recent large, randomized controlled trial demonstrated the efficacy of early adenotonsillectomy in improving behavior, quality of life, and polysomnographic features of childhood OSAS.[10] Although most patients with OSAS will undergo surgery, not all pediatric patients with OSAS are appropriate surgical candidates. In addition, some patients continue to be symptomatic and have polysomnographic evidence of residual OSAS after adenotonsillectomy; risk factors include severe preoperative OSAS, obesity, neuromuscular disorders characterized by hypotonia, and craniofacial abnormalities.[24–26] These patients may be candidates for positive airway pressure (PAP) therapy.[27]

MECHANISM OF ACTION OF PAP

PAP is a noninvasive method of treating OSAS, and is the most common treatment modality in adults. The basic mechanism involves it delivering intraluminal airway pressure that is above the critical closing pressure of the airway to overcome dynamic obstruction by stenting the airway open.[28,29] This positive pressure is generated by an air compressor in the continuous PAP (CPAP) machine, and is transmitted to the patient's airway through a single conduit that connects with the patient via a variety of interfaces, including nasal pillows, nasal masks (**Fig. 1**), and full-face masks. The device continually adjusts its output to the patient's breathing pattern to maintain a constant pressure. A fixed leak valve is positioned near the mask to prevent rebreathing of carbon dioxide. **Fig. 1** shows a typical PAP apparatus.

It must be noted that it is not the movement of air but rather the pressure generated and maintained through the airway that prevents obstructive events. Selection of an appropriately sized mask that provides a snug fit devoid of air leaks is central to maintenance of positive pressure throughout the system. Mask straps, cushions around the interface, and forehead spacers facilitate mask fit and comfort.

Contemporary CPAP devices have evolved in both size and function, with devices becoming more portable and technologically advanced. Most CPAP machines available today are equipped with data-storage capabilities, digitally recording the number of apnea events and air leaks over time. Data can be downloaded from the machine during follow-up, and serve as an objective measure of CPAP usage to provide feedback to the patient and family to aid in improving adherence. In addition, the incorporation of a humidifier in PAP devices has been demonstrated in adults to decrease drying of the nasal mucosa that can lead to nasal congestion, dryness, and epistaxis, and to increase adherence.[30,31]

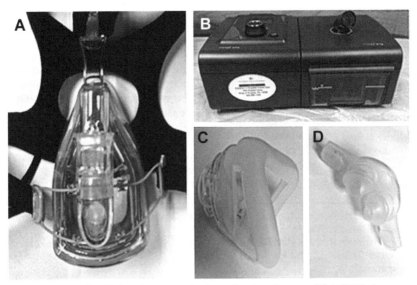

Fig. 1. (*A*) A full-face CPAP mask with headgear attached to a forehead spacer. (*B*) A CPAP air compressor machine with humidifier. (*C*) A nasal CPAP mask. (*D*) A nasal CPAP device with nasal pillows.

EFFICACY OF PAP FOR THE TREATMENT OF CHILDHOOD OSAS

Although it should be noted that the use of home CPAP for children weighing less than 40 lb (18 kg) or younger than 7 years has not been approved by the US Food and Drug Administration, extensive clinical experience and numerous studies have demonstrated CPAP to be safe and efficacious in children of all ages, including infants.[32–34] Marcus and colleagues[27] demonstrated PAP therapy (both CPAP and bilevel PAP [BPAP]) to be effective in improving respiratory parameters in pediatric patients aged 2 to 16 years with OSAS, with highly significant improvements in both the apnea-hypopnea index (AHI; number of apneas and hypopneas per hour of sleep) ($P = .003$) and oxyhemoglobin saturation nadir ($P = .001$) 6 months after initiating PAP therapy.[27] These results were accompanied by significant improvements in subjective parental assessment of sleepiness, snoring, and difficulty breathing during sleep.

CHALLENGES OF PAP ADHERENCE

Benefit from CPAP therapy is predicated on a snugly fit mask that can maintain positive pressure to stent the upper airway. Adherence with the device can be difficult, especially for children with developmental delays, anxiety, or other behavioral problems. These children often verbally and physically resist the caregiver's efforts to put on the mask. Consequently, they develop conditioned anxiety because of poorly fitting equipment and repeated association of the sight, sound, and sensation of CPAP with discomfort from the mask, physiologic arousal from struggling, or both.[35]

When treatment failure occurs in the course of OSAS treatment with CPAP, adherence is the major cause, accounting for up to 92% in one study.[32] Earlier studies on the efficacy of CPAP in childhood OSAS used subjective self-report and parent-report measures of CPAP usage, and reported a high rate of adherence.[32,36] More recently, usage recordings by the CPAP machine, which can be digitally downloaded, have enabled objective assessments of adherence and have demonstrated CPAP adherence to be frequently suboptimal. **Table 1** summarizes studies investigating CPAP adherence in children.

In a randomized double-blind trial comparing the efficacy and adherence of CPAP and BPAP in PAP-naïve children with OSAS, intention-to-treat analysis that included 8 of 29 patients who failed to return for CPAP usage downloads found adherence for all participants to be suboptimal, at an average usage of 3.8 ± 3.3 hours per night.[27] Another study by O'Donnell and colleagues[37] reported similar findings of suboptimal adherence, with mean usage of 4.7 hours per night. These results are similar to the findings of a group of Australian investigators who also found a mean CPAP use of 4.7 hours in their study evaluating patterns of CPAP adherence during the first 3 months of treatment in children.[38] However, it should be noted that although these numbers are close to or higher than the adult criteria for satisfactory CPAP adherence[39] (ie, at least 4 hours/night on 70% of nights), children have a longer sleep duration than adults, and thus thresholds for "adequate" levels of adherence may actually be higher. Furthermore, a study by Marcus and colleagues[40] suggested that longer duration of CPAP use (mean minutes used per night) correlates inversely with Epworth Sleepiness Scale scores.

It should also be noted that data collected in the context and controlled setting of a study may not reflect typical levels of adherence in practice settings, in which monitoring, feedback, and support levels are likely to be less intense. This aspect represents a particular challenge for clinicians caring for children with OSAS in clinical practice. Even in an experimental setting, one study reported a dropout rate of 24% (7 of 29) during the course of an investigation that provided free equipment and comprehensive social and technical support.[41] It can be theorized that the reluctance to continue with CPAP treatment in the clinical setting, where resources may be limited, is even more prevalent.

FACTORS INFLUENCING CPAP ADHERENCE

Literature from studies on adult CPAP adherence identified categories of factors that influence or predict adherence to CPAP use: (1) disease characteristics; (2) patient characteristics; (3) treatment titration procedures; (4) technological device factors and side effects; and (5) psychological and social factors. A summary of these factors and their relationship to the course of CPAP treatment is summarized in **Table 2**.[42]

Although these categories provide a framework to better understand patients' decisions to adhere to CPAP treatment, one cannot simply extrapolate and assume that these factors are important in the pediatric population. Several retrospective and observational studies also implicate some of these factors in poor CPAP adherence in the pediatric population. However, although only a few prospective studies,[43,44] discussed herein, are

Table 1
Summary of select studies investigating CPAP adherence in children

Authors, Ref. Year	Population	Age	OSAS Characteristics	Associated Conditions	Measure of Adherence	Findings
DiFeo et al,[43] 2012	N = 56 children and their parents 68% male 59% African American 36% Caucasian	2–16 y	AHI 19 ± 16/h Naïve to CPAP	71% obese 23% with neurodevelopmental disabilities 20% with genetic syndromes	Usage data from machine (at 1 and 3 mo)	Average use 3 ± 3 h per night after first month, 2.8 ± 2.7 h on third month Greatest predictor of use was maternal education Older, typically developing African American youth with low social support had poor adherence
Simon et al,[44] 2012	N = 51 children and their parents 51% male 51% non-Hispanic Caucasian 37% African American 64% had Medicaid	8–17 y	Average AHI 17/h Average CPAP use of 22.9 mo	73.5% overweight/ obese	Usage data from machine	Poor adherence with average use of 3.35 h per night Questionnaire developed was able to identify specific barriers to CPAP
Marcus et al,[41] 2006	N = 29 children 72% male 51% African American	2–16 y	Newly diagnosed OSAS	65% obese 10% craniofacial abnormalities 34% systolic hypertension	Parental report and usage data from machine for 6 mo	Average use 3.8 ± 3.3 h per night 9 dropouts Parental report overestimated actual use No difference in adherence between CPAP and BPAP

			Median AHI = 11.3	78% with comorbidity	Usage data from machine	Average use 6.3 h per night
O'Donnell et al,[37] 2006	N = 50 children	Mean 10 ± 5.1 y 66% male	Median AHI = 11.3	78% with comorbidity	Usage data from machine	Average use 6.3 h per night
Koontz et al,[35] 2003	N = 20 children 55% African American 30% Caucasian	1–17 y	Nonadherent children referred by physicians	45% with some degree of developmental delay	Usage data from machine	3 groups: 1. Consultation (usage 8.58 h/night) 2. Consultation with behavior therapy (usage 5.88 h/night) 3. No consultation/behavior therapy (usage 0.67 h/night)
Massa et al,[36] 2002	N = 66 children 59% male	Infant to 19 y	All moderate to severe OSAS (AHI >5 per hour)	35% craniosynostosis syndromes 9.1% isolated facial defects 6.1% obese 3% trisomy 21 3% cerebral palsy	Parental report	67.7% report good adherence (uses every night and all night long) CPAP tolerated by 86%
Marcus et al,[17] 1994	N = 94 children 64% male	2 wk to 19 y	—	27% obese 25% craniofacial abnormalities 13% trisomy 21	Parental report	12.7% with inadequate adherence

Abbreviations: AHI, apnea-hypopnea index; BPAP, bilevel positive airway pressure; CPAP, continuous positive airway pressure; OSAS, obstructive sleep apnea syndrome.
Data from Refs.[17,35–37,41,43,44]

Table 2
Factors that influence on CPAP adherence in adults

Factor	Relationship to Course of Treatment		
	Pre-CPAP Exposure	Initial CPAP Exposure	Home CPAP Treatment
Disease and patient characteristics	Disease severity Sleepiness Upper airway patency Race Socioeconomic status	Depression Mood Personality type	Depression Mood Personality type
Treatment titration procedure	—	Autotitrating CPAP	—
Technological device factors and side effects	Claustrophobia	Heated humidification	Heated humidification
Psychological and social factors	Disease- and treatment-specific knowledge	Disease- and treatment-specific knowledge	Disease- and treatment-specific knowledge Decisional balance Active coping style Disease-specific risk perception

Abbreviation: CPAP, continuous positive airway pressure.

Adapted from Sawyer AM, Gooneratne NS, Marcus CL, et al. A systematic review of CPAP adherence across age groups: clinical and empiric insights for developing CPAP adherence interventions. Sleep Med Rev 2011;15(6):345; with permission.

available, these seem to demonstrate a different profile of factors from those shown to predict poor adherence in adults.

Psychosocial Factors

One prospective study collected data potentially pertaining to CPAP adherence and correlated these with objective CPAP adherence data. In their cohort of 56 children aged 2 to16 years, DiFeo and colleagues[43] evaluated patient characteristics (obesity, race, gender), disease characteristics (severity of OSAS as evidence by AHI), child characteristics (presence/absence of developmental delay and attention-deficit/hyperactivity disorder), CPAP-related factors (CPAP pressure and nasal symptoms), and psychosocial factors (maternal education, social support). Financial/insurance barriers were controlled for by providing all of the participants with free equipment and treatment.[43] Their analysis revealed that the greatest predictor of CPAP use was maternal education ($r = 0.290$, $P = .033$ for mean hours used per night). Disease-specific factors such as polysomnographic measures and symptoms of excessive daytime sleepiness, which predict CPAP adherence in the adult population, did not significantly correlate with poor CPAP use, nor was there predictive value found in clinical factors such as CPAP pressure and nasal symptoms. The investigators postulated that higher maternal education

provided better parental understanding of the consequences of OSAS and the importance of treatment adherence.

DiFeo and colleagues[43] also found the Medical Outcomes Study Social Support (MOSS) questionnaire, a measure of family social support, to be somewhat predictive of CPAP adherence, though not as strongly as maternal education. This finding suggests that a combination of caregiver (in this case mothers) knowledge and social support are both important to adherence in children. Several empirical investigations have found that patients' level of adherence is positively associated with their motivation to achieve or maintain good health. Cobb and Jones[45] suggested that social support encompasses: (1) the supportive behavior of individuals family and friends; (2) the nature of the social network surrounding individuals; and (3) the individual's perceptions of the support provided by their family and friends. However, social support may also exert a stressful influence on the patient when the level of support is perceived as threatening to the patient's autonomy.[46] This influence is likely to be of greatest importance with adolescent patients.

Patients' Characteristics

In the aforementioned prospective study that evaluated risk factors for pediatric CPAP adherence, DiFeo and colleagues[43] also found that certain patient characteristics predicted poor CPAP adherence. African American children, independent of socioeconomic status, were less likely to be adherent to CPAP than children of other races. This finding mirrors observations found in adult CPAP adherence literature.[47] Older children, particularly adolescents, were also less likely to adhere to CPAP therapy, which is consistent with data from studies of adherence to other pediatric medical regimens (see later discussion).[48–50]

Device Factors

Most studies have shown that the type of CPAP device used does not affect adherence, suggesting that adherence is affected by general factors more than by device-specific or disease-specific factors. However, one pediatric study showed that full-face masks were associated with lower adherence than nasal masks.[37] Studies in both children and adults comparing different types of pressure delivery, such as BPAP or C-Flex/BiFlex (which deliver a slight decrease in pressure during early expiration and/or inspiration), have had mixed results, but have generally not shown an improvement in adherence in comparison with standard CPAP.[41,51,52]

Factors Affecting Adherence in Adolescents

Studies on adherence to other medical regimens for the treatment of asthma, epilepsy, and diabetes have shown poor adherence in adolescents.[53,54] In their review of factors influencing adherence to medical treatments, Fotheringham and Sawyer[46] observed lower adherence in adolescents than in adults. These investigators argue that poor adherence may be due to the struggle for greater autonomy at home, and reflects rebellion against the regimens' control over patients' lives.

There is a paucity of data describing CPAP adherence in adolescents. Prashad and colleagues[55] investigated CPAP adherence in 21 adolescents using qualitative semistructured interviews that explored issues of stress, parenting style, family structure and organization, behavioral and emotional problems, knowledge of OSAS, and benefits of CPAP, combined with usage data from the CPAP machine. Their qualitative results found that patients/families with high CPAP usage had stable family structure, high knowledge of CPAP, free communication between parent and adolescent, motivation from a desire to please the caregiver, and an "authoritative parenting style"[56] whereby children are encouraged to inquire about rules to fully understand them. In this context, parents explained the importance of CPAP use and

gave adolescents the choice to use CPAP or not. Adherence was also higher in patients who were prescribed CPAP before adolescence. This finding was postulated to be related to the longer opportunity for CPAP to become a part of the patient's routine when it is prescribed at a younger age, instead of in adolescence when issues of rebellion and emerging autonomy may prove challenging. It was concluded that health education and family involvement are important components in promoting CPAP adherence, and that support strategies should be tailored to the individual and take into account the developmental process of adolescence.

OVERCOMING BARRIERS TO ADHERENCE
Child/Parent Engagement

Successful promotion of CPAP adherence infers addressing child/parent engagement in the initial acceptance of CPAP. Some barriers to this include preconceived notions about CPAP, and outcome expectations incongruent to that of the treating physician and staff.[57] Determination of the child's and parent's preexisting attitudes toward CPAP is an important first step, and functions to dispel disbeliefs and tailor patient education on outcome expectations. Central to this process of engaging the child and the parent is maintenance of a positive and supportive approach by everyone involved. Such an approach is especially important in children with complex medical problems, for whom gradual CPAP exposure in a supportive setting and anticipatory guidance for troubleshooting may be particularly important.[42]

Identification of Specific Barriers

To improve adherence, it is vital to identify specific barriers to adherence that both families and patients themselves experience. A significant portion of the literature on adherence has focused predominantly on the concerns of the patients' family alone.[58] To address this gap, Simon and colleagues[44] constructed a psychometric questionnaire to evaluate child and family barriers to CPAP adherence. The Adherence Barriers to CPAP Questionnaire (ABCQ) included 31 questions developed across several conceptually derived domains including side effects, time management, health care provider relationships, equipment concerns, and family support, to name a few. The ABCQ demonstrated excellent reliability and validity, and correlated with objective adherence rates. Having a greater amount of barriers identified on ABCQ was associated with poorer rates of adherence for both parent ($r = -0.44$, $P = .002$) and the child ($r = -0.44$, $P = .002$). **Table 3** summarizes the most frequently endorsed

Table 3
Most frequently endorsed barriers to CPAP reported on the ABCQ

Parent-Report Item (% Agree/Strongly Agree)		Child-Report Item (% Agree/Strongly Agree)	
Does not use when away from home	45.1	Does not use when away from home	47.0
Child not feeling well	44.0	Just want to forget about OSAS	43.1
Forgets	39.2	Not feeling well	42.0
Child does not feel like using CPAP	30.0	Forgets	39.2
Child just wants to forget about OSAS	23.6	No one helps to use CPAP at night	31.4
Child embarrassed about using CPAP	22.0	Embarrassed about using CPAP	29.4

Abbreviations: ABCQ, adherence barriers to CPAP questionnaire; CPAP, continuous positive airway pressure; OSAS, obstructive sleep apnea syndrome.

Adapted from Simon SL, Duncan CL, Janicke DM, et al. Barriers to treatment of paediatric obstructive sleep apnoea: development of the adherence barriers to continuous positive airway pressure (CPAP) questionnaire. Sleep Med 2012;13(2):172–7; with permission.

Table 4
Desensitization procedure for infants and school-aged children

Daytime Practice	Nighttime Practice

Introducing the mask
  The child and parent play together with the mask and machine. The parent puts the PAP on a stuffed animal, doll, themselves, etc
  Place the mask (not attached to the hose/machine) on your child's face for 5 s
  Place the mask (not attached to the hose/machine) on your child's face for 10 s
  Place the mask (not attached to the hose/machine) on your child's face for 1 min
  Place the mask on your child's face and connect the headgear on *both* sides for 1 min
  Repeat above step, slowly increasing the amount of time your child wears the mask and headgear each practice session
	Adjusting to the sounds at night
	  While your child is going through desensitization practice during the day, begin turning on the PAP machine at night without attaching it to your child so he/she can get used to the noise

Turning on the air
  Place the mask and headgear on your child; attach the hose to the mask and to the machine, and turn the air on for 5 s
  Repeat above step, slowly increasing the amount of time each practice session
Wearing the mask with airflow while lying down
  Have your child lie down on the bed or couch. Place the mask (attached to the hose and both sides of the cap) on your child's face for 5 min
  Have your child lie down on the bed or couch. Place the mask (attached to the hose and both sides of the cap) on your child's face for 10 min
  Have your child lie down on the bed or couch. Place the mask (attached to the hose and both sides of the cap) for your child's face or 15 min
	Making PAP part of your child's bedtime routine
	  Add PAP to your child's bedtime routine. Have your child try to fall asleep after you place the mask (attached to the hose on both sides of the cap) on the face and the air is turned on for 15 min
	  Continue nightly until your child is able to fall asleep with PAP. If your child cannot fall asleep with PAP, do 15 min of practice
	  Continue daytime practice and bedtime practice until your child is able to fall asleep with PAP on and sleep with it for most of the night. Replace PAP at night if it falls off or is removed

Abbreviation: PAP, positive airway pressure.

Adapted from The Children's Hospital of Philadelphia. CPAP education: noninvasive ventilation for infants and children. 2013. Available at: http://www.chop.edu/service/sleep-center/cpap-education/non-invasive-ventilation-for-infants-and-children.html. Accessed November 25, 2013; with permission.

barriers to CPAP reported. The ABCQ represents the first tool specifically to assess specific barriers to CPAP, but further investigation is needed to determine its utility as a measure of treatment outcomes.

Initial Acceptance

An unpleasant initial exposure to CPAP has been observed to lead to a prolonged period of treatment rejection from both child and caregiver.[57] Patients with tactile aversions (eg, children with developmental delays) are particularly challenging because they are not typically accepting of the mask at the time of initial presentation. Families and medical practitioners must be prepared to invest substantial time and patience toward successfully initiating and maintaining CPAP therapy.

Overcoming the child's aversion to CPAP may require desensitization procedures that allow the child to slowly habituate by gradual exposure to the mask and machine (ie, operant conditioning). An example would be to divide the procedures into daytime and nighttime practices in an attempt to establish CPAP as part of the child's routine activities.[59] This approach is further detailed in **Table 4**. Each practice session should start with an enjoyable, calming activity so the child begins to associate CPAP with positive experiences. The child should be offered small rewards such

as stickers or a prize each time he or she is successful with the practice session, in addition to a verbal praise when the child complies with the parental request. Any negative behaviors such as crying or yelling are ignored. For older children or adolescents, a token economy can be implemented, designed to increase desirable behavior and decrease undesirable behavior with the use of tokens, such as stickers or check marks. The child should receive a sticker immediately after displaying desirable behavior (eg, complying with a request to put the CPAP mask on for designated amount of time). The stickers are collected (or counted up on a chart) and later exchanged for a meaningful object or privilege. Emphasis is placed on practice, patience, and persistence for the overall implementation of CPAP. The goal is to avoid struggles and negative interactions around CPAP, and to implement CPAP in the least stressful way possible for children and parents.

The location where CPAP initiation occurs has also been observed to have an effect on adherence to therapy. Ramirez and colleagues[60] evaluated long-term adherence to CPAP among 62 children with OSAS who were followed in a pediatric CPAP/noninvasive unit. A high level of adherence was observed in patients who initiated CPAP and followed up in the unit. The investigators postulated that the high level of adherence may have been due to the availability of a dedicated team

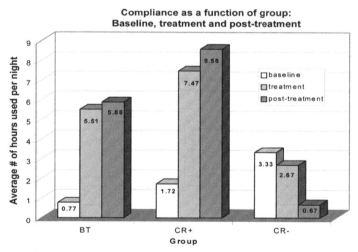

Fig. 2. Results of CPAP adherence strategies in a group of children referred for behavioral counseling for poor CPAP adherence. Subjects were divided into 3 groups: BT received consultation and recommendations plus a course of behavior therapy; CR+ received a 1.5-hour consultation and recommendation session; CR− underwent a consultation and behavior therapy was recommended, but the family did not follow up. The y-axis shows the average number of hours per night of CPAP use. The hours of use are further subdivided into baseline, during treatment, and posttreatment values. Seventy-five percent of children who received behavior intervention (CR+ and BT groups) tolerated CPAP successfully (P<.5 for CR+ vs CR− group; other comparisons were not significant). (*Adapted from* Koontz KL, Slifer KJ, Cataldo MD, et al. Improving pediatric compliance with positive airway pressure therapy: the impact of behavioral intervention. Sleep 2003;26(8):1012; with permission.)

that provided positive and continuous support for the patient and family from CPAP initiation through follow-up. However, most patients can successfully undergo CPAP initiation in the outpatient setting.

Behavioral Intervention

Behavioral conditioning may be a useful tool to help achieve CPAP acceptance. Koontz and colleagues[35] studied 20 children with OSAS, aged 1 to 17 years, who were referred from their respective primary physicians for CPAP nonadherence. Patients and their guardians were then allowed to self-select into 1 of 3 treatment arms: (1) behavior therapy; (2) behavior consultation and recommendation uptake; (3) behavior consultation without recommendation uptake. Before assignments into their respective treatment arms, all children and their guardians attended a behavior consultation with trained staff. This consultation sought to identify individual information about the child's preferences and dislikes to generate recommendations. Results of the study showed that patients in both behavior therapy (75%) and behavior consultation with recommendation uptake (100%) had a statistically significantly heavier CPAP use than those in the behavior consultation group without recommendation uptake (0%). A graphic representation of the results is shown in **Fig. 2.**

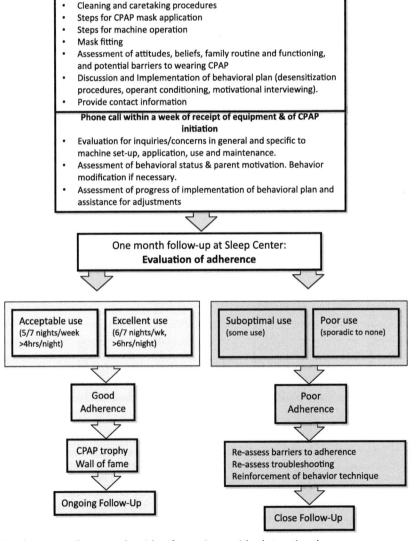

Fig. 3. Example of a CPAP adherence algorithm for patients with obstructive sleep apnea.

This retrospective and descriptive interventional study suggests that both brief behavior consultations and extensive behavioral therapy may offer effective and relatively inexpensive interventions for CPAP adherence.

Side Effects

Similar to any form of treatment, CPAP has associated side effects that may have a negative impact on adherence if unaddressed. Nasal symptoms are the most common side effect, caused by the drying effects of CPAP by altering nasal mucosa and impeding mucociliary clearance.[30,61] This symptom can be ameliorated with a heated humidifier, maintenance of clean equipment, and, in some cases, intranasal steroids, saline, antihistamines, montelukast, or other treatments.[31,62] Skin irritation and even ulceration can occur from a tight-fitting mask or accumulation of skin oils and debris from poor mask maintenance; rarely, allergies to the mask may occur.[57] A properly fitted mask and daily cleaning of the equipment is thus integral to CPAP adherence. Central apnea at high pressures can be a complication of CPAP use in some children because of an active Hering-Breuer reflex.[63] Switching from CPAP to BPAP with a backup rate addresses this problem.

AN EXAMPLE OF A CLINICAL APPROACH

The Sleep Center at The Children's Hospital of Philadelphia (CHOP) is a tertiary referral center for children with a broad range of sleep disorders (**Fig. 3**, see **Table 4**). The center comprises a multidisciplinary team of sleep physicians, behavioral psychologists, respiratory therapists, and nurses, collaborating to provide comprehensive evaluation and management of patients with various sleep disorders, including OSAS. A general description of the CHOP PAP protocol as a model of care follows.

The sleep physician's role in the initial CPAP visit is to educate the family about OSAS, its pathophysiology, complications, and the importance of treating it. The basic mechanism of how CPAP works and side effects that might be encountered are also discussed. The respiratory therapist and nurses present different types of mask interfaces from which the family/patient can choose. The patient is encouraged to try on several masks to determine which is the most comfortable (**Fig. 4**). Having the patient and family involved in choosing the mask offers them an opportunity to increase a sense of control in a situation where they may feel a loss of control. The psychologist assesses the patient's and caregiver's attitudes and beliefs about CPAP, potential barriers to using CPAP, in

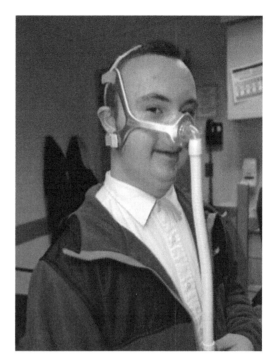

Fig. 4. A patient with trisomy 21 trying on a nasal mask during a CPAP initiation visit.

addition to family functioning and patient and family routines. He or she then discusses behavioral techniques (eg, mask desensitization, operant conditioning) to help improve adherence, as well as strategies to implement CPAP into the specific patient's daily routine. For example, for a family whose household is chaotic or whose child does not have a "typical routine," the psychologist and family may together develop a specific evening and bedtime routine that ends with putting on the CPAP.

For an adolescent, it may be beneficial to discuss a division of responsibilities between the adolescent and caregiver to reduce feelings in both parties of being overburdened. A caregiver may agree to remind the adolescent to get his or her CPAP ready before bed and to help with the deeper weekly cleaning of the equipment, while the adolescent agrees to be responsible for putting the CPAP on each night and participate in the daily care of the equipment (eg, pouring water out of the humidifier, rinsing the humidifier, tubing, and mask each day, and setting out to air dry in the morning). This strategy aims to respect and improve the autonomy and responsibility of the adolescent while providing the necessary support he or she likely needs in adhering to a medical intervention without a sense of being nagged.

A durable medical equipment representative also meets with the family to discuss machine operation, maintenance, and troubleshooting, and to provide equipment for the family to take home that day. At the end of the visit, it is verified that the family is given a network of support by providing contact information for them to call in case of further inquiry. This process is spearheaded by the CPAP coordinator (a position split between a respiratory therapist and psychologist)

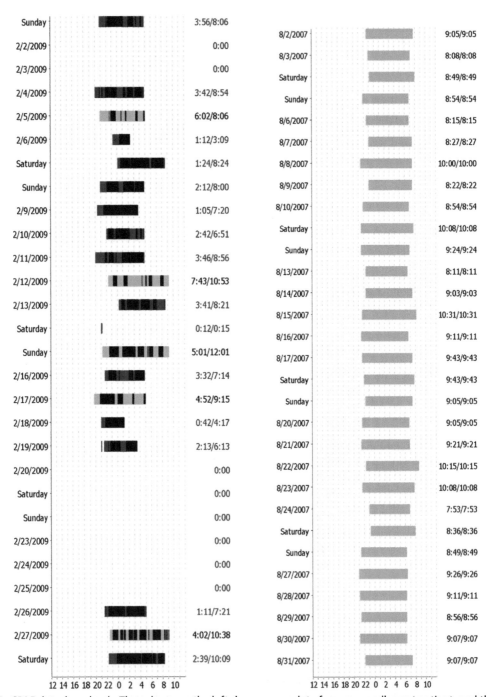

Fig. 5. CPAP data downloads. The column on the left shows usage data from a nonadherent patient, and the column on the right is from an adherent patient. The x-axis shows 24-hour clock time and the left y-axis shows the date. CPAP use for 4 hours or more is shown in green, less than 4 hours in red; air leak is shown in black. Corresponding numbers are shown on the right y-axis. Air leak may be due to the mask being damaged, fitting poorly, or being off the face when the air compressor is turned on.

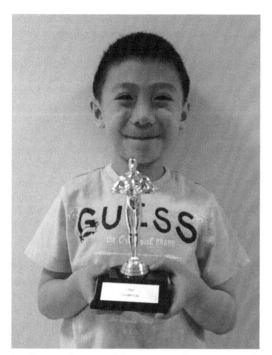

Fig. 6. A patient receiving a CPAP champion trophy for good adherence.

to provide an organized channel for subsequent clinic follow-up. A CPAP titration polysomnogram is typically not performed until the child is tolerating CPAP set at a low pressure at home.

Within a week, a phone call is made by a CPAP coordinator to check adherence and to troubleshoot any problems such as device issues or CPAP side effects, as well as to assess behavioral implementation concerns or barriers. If behavioral concerns exist or persist, the psychologist follows up by phone regularly. The respiratory therapist and nurses also provide phone support for technical or side effects and medical concerns as needed. Patients are encouraged to follow up at the clinic after 1 month, at which time adherence is assessed. The CPAP machine's usage data is downloaded to provide an objective measure of the patient's adherence. The results are then discussed with the patient and family, who are shown a visual representation of the usage (**Fig. 5**). Those who have good adherence are given an incentive CPAP trophy (when developmentally appropriate) (**Fig. 6**) and have their picture posted on the "CPAP Hall of Fame." Patients with poor adherence are reassessed by the team for specific barriers to adherence such as troubleshooting machine problems, issues with the mask fit or putting it on correctly, or behavioral barriers. Adolescents may need help troubleshooting simple issues, such as finding an electrical outlet near

their bed, developing a plan to take their machine with them when staying overnight at relatives' or friends' homes, or setting an alert on their phone to remind them to put on their mask at night. For all patients, technical support and behavioral reinforcement is provided, with close follow-up thereafter. Children are seen on a regular basis, with the frequency of their clinic visits depending on their age, severity of medical condition, and CPAP adherence.

In almost all cases, CPAP is implemented in an outpatient setting. Occasionally a family (typically with an infant, toddler, or developmentally delayed child) is unable to implement a desensitization program, and a short 2- to 4-week intervention with home nursing is implemented. This approach often breaks the cycle of CPAP refusal, anxiety, and frustration, and demonstrates to the family that the child can tolerate CPAP. Typically parents are able to continue implementing CPAP at the end of the nursing intervention. Rarely, patients are admitted to an inpatient unit when all other measures fail.

SUMMARY

CPAP is a safe and effective treatment for children with OSAS that has many beneficial effects. The major limiting factor for successful treatment with CPAP is adherence. Psychosocial factors and patient characteristics are the main predictors of poor adherence, with low maternal education being the strongest. Managing suboptimal adherence entails engaging and educating the child and parent about CPAP. This approach involves discussing preexisting attitudes, outcome expectations, and side effects, in addition to providing constant support from a dedicated team. More intensive cognitive-behavioral interventions may prove useful in overcoming poor CPAP adherence in complex cases.

ACKNOWLEDGMENTS

The authors would like to thank the Children's Hospital of Philadelphia CPAP team for their dedication to patients and their families.

REFERENCES

1. Marcus CL, Brooks LJ, Draper KA, et al. Diagnosis and management of childhood obstructive sleep apnea syndrome. Pediatrics 2012;130(3):e714–55.
2. Bixler EO, Vgontzas AN, Lin HM, et al. Sleep disordered breathing in children in a general population sample: prevalence and risk factors. Sleep 2009; 32(6):731–6.

3. Li AM, So HK, Au CT, et al. Epidemiology of obstructive sleep apnoea syndrome in Chinese children: a two-phase community study. Thorax 2010;65(11):991–7.

4. O'Brien LM, Holbrook CR, Mervis CB, et al. Sleep and neurobehavioral characteristics of 5- to 7-year-old children with parentally reported symptoms of attention-deficit/hyperactivity disorder. Pediatrics 2003;111(3):554–63.

5. Chervin RD, Ruzicka DL, Giordani BJ, et al. Sleep-disordered breathing, behavior, and cognition in children before and after adenotonsillectomy. Pediatrics 2006;117(4):e769–78.

6. Beebe DW, Ris MD, Kramer ME, et al. The association between sleep disordered breathing, academic grades, and cognitive and behavioral functioning among overweight subjects during middle to late childhood. Sleep 2010;33(11): 1447–56.

7. Beebe DW, Byars KC. Adolescents with obstructive sleep apnea adhere poorly to positive airway pressure (PAP), but PAP users show improved attention and school performance. PLoS One 2011;6(3): e16924.

8. Kurnatowski P, Putyński L, Lapienis M, et al. Neurocognitive abilities in children with adenotonsillar hypertrophy. Int J Pediatr Otorhinolaryngol 2006; 70(3):419–24.

9. Barnes ME, Gozal D, Molfese DL. Attention in children with obstructive sleep apnoea: an event-related potentials study. Sleep Med 2012;13(4): 368–77.

10. Marcus CL, Moore RH, Rosen CL, et al. A randomized trial of adenotonsillectomy for childhood sleep apnea. N Engl J Med 2013;368(25): 2366–76.

11. Marcus CL, Greene MG, Carroll JL. Blood pressure in children with obstructive sleep apnea. Am J Respir Crit Care Med 1998;157(4 Pt 1):1098–103.

12. Amin RS, Kimball TR, Bean JA, et al. Left ventricular hypertrophy and abnormal ventricular geometry in children and adolescents with obstructive sleep apnea. Am J Respir Crit Care Med 2002;165(10): 1395–9.

13. Duman D, Naiboglu B, Esen HS, et al. Impaired right ventricular function in adenotonsillar hypertrophy. Int J Cardiovasc Imaging 2008;24(3): 261–7.

14. Hunt CE, Brouillette RT. Abnormalities of breathing control and airway maintenance in infants and children as a cause of cor pulmonale. Pediatr Cardiol 1982;3(3):249–56.

15. Kelly A, Dougherty S, Cucchiara A, et al. Catecholamines, adiponectin, and insulin resistance as measured by HOMA in children with obstructive sleep apnea. Sleep 2010;33(9):1185–91.

16. Deboer MD, Mendoza JP, Liu L, et al. Increased systemic inflammation overnight correlates with insulin resistance among children evaluated for obstructive sleep apnea. Sleep Breath 2012; 16(2):349–54.

17. Marcus CL, Carroll JL, Koerner CB, et al. Determinants of growth in children with the obstructive sleep apnea syndrome. J Pediatr 1994;125(4): 556–62.

18. Mezzanotte WS, Tangel DJ, White DP. Influence of sleep onset on upper-airway muscle activity in apnea patients versus normal controls. Am J Respir Crit Care Med 1996;153(6 Pt 1):1880–7.

19. Kulnis R, Nelson S, Strohl K, et al. Cephalometric assessment of snoring and nonsnoring children. Chest 2000;118(3):596–603.

20. Brooks LJ, Stephens BM, Bacevice AM. Adenoid size is related to severity but not the number of episodes of obstructive apnea in children. J Pediatr 1998;132(4):682–6.

21. Shintani T, Asakura K, Kataura A. Evaluation of the role of adenotonsillar hypertrophy and facial morphology in children with obstructive sleep apnea. ORL J Otorhinolaryngol Relat Spec 1997; 59(5):286–91.

22. Marcus CL. Obstructive sleep apnea syndrome: differences between children and adults. Sleep 2000;23(Suppl 4):S140–1.

23. Arens R, McDonough JM, Costarino AT, et al. Magnetic resonance imaging of the upper airway structure of children with obstructive sleep apnea syndrome. Am J Respir Crit Care Med 2001; 164(4):698–703.

24. Smith DF, Benke JR, Yaster S, et al. A pilot staging system to predict persistent obstructive sleep apnea in children following adenotonsillectomy. Laryngoscope 2013;123(7):1817–22.

25. Mitchell RB, Kelly J. Outcome of adenotonsillectomy for obstructive sleep apnea in obese and normal-weight children. Otolaryngol Head Neck Surg 2007;137(1):43–8.

26. Suen JS, Arnold JE, Brooks LJ. Adenotonsillectomy for treatment of obstructive sleep apnea in children. Arch Otolaryngol Head Neck Surg 1995; 121(5):525–30.

27. Marcus CL, Beck SE, Traylor J, et al. Randomized, double-blind clinical trial of two different modes of positive airway pressure therapy on adherence and efficacy in children. J Clin Sleep Med 2012; 8(1):37–42.

28. Marcus CL, McColley SA, Carroll JL, et al. Upper airway collapsibility in children with obstructive sleep apnea syndrome. J Appl Physiol (1985) 1994;77(2):918–24.

29. Smith PL, Wise RA, Gold AR, et al. Upper airway pressure-flow relationships in obstructive

sleep apnea. J Appl Physiol (1985) 1988;64(2): 789–95.

30. Pepin JL, Leger P, Veale D, et al. Side effects of nasal continuous positive airway pressure in sleep apnea syndrome. Study of 193 patients in two French sleep centers. Chest 1995;107(2):375–81.

31. Massie CA, Hart RW, Peralez K, et al. Effects of humidification on nasal symptoms and compliance in sleep apnea patients using continuous positive airway pressure. Chest 1999;116(2):403–8.

32. Marcus CL, Ward SL, Mallory GB, et al. Use of nasal continuous positive airway pressure as treatment of childhood obstructive sleep apnea. J Pediatr 1995;127(1):88–94.

33. McNamara F, Sullivan CE. Obstructive sleep apnea in infants and its management with nasal continuous positive airway pressure. Chest 1999;116(1):10–6.

34. Downey R 3rd, Perkin RM, MacQuarrie J. Nasal continuous positive airway pressure use in children with obstructive sleep apnea younger than 2 years of age. Chest 2000;117(6):1608–12.

35. Koontz KL, Slifer KJ, Cataldo MD, et al. Improving pediatric compliance with positive airway pressure therapy: the impact of behavioral intervention. Sleep 2003;26(8):1010–5.

36. Massa F, Gonsalez S, Laverty A, et al. The use of nasal continuous positive airway pressure to treat obstructive sleep apnoea. Arch Dis Child 2002; 87(5):438–43.

37. O'Donnell AR, Bjornson CL, Bohn SG, et al. Compliance rates in children using noninvasive continuous positive airway pressure. Sleep 2006; 29(5):651–8.

38. Nixon GM, Mihai R, Verginis N, et al. Patterns of continuous positive airway pressure adherence during the first 3 months of treatment in children. J Pediatr 2011;159(5):802–7.

39. Pepin JL, Krieger J, Rodenstein D, et al. Effective compliance during the first 3 months of continuous positive airway pressure. A European prospective study of 121 patients. Am J Respir Crit Care Med 1999;160(4):1124–9.

40. Marcus CL, Radcliffe J, Konstantinopoulou S, et al. Effects of positive airway pressure therapy on neurobehavioral outcomes in children with obstructive sleep apnea. Am J Respir Crit Care Med 2012; 185(9):998–1003.

41. Marcus CL, Rosen G, Ward SL, et al. Adherence to and effectiveness of positive airway pressure therapy in children with obstructive sleep apnea. Pediatrics 2006;117(3):e442–51.

42. Sawyer AM, Gooneratne NS, Marcus CL, et al. A systematic review of CPAP adherence across age groups: clinical and empiric insights for developing CPAP adherence interventions. Sleep Med Rev 2011;15(6):343–56.

43. DiFeo N, Meltzer LJ, Beck SE, et al. Predictors of positive airway pressure therapy adherence in children: a prospective study. J Clin Sleep Med 2012; 8(3):279–86.

44. Simon SL, Duncan CL, Janicke DM, et al. Barriers to treatment of paediatric obstructive sleep apnoea: development of the adherence barriers to continuous positive airway pressure (CPAP) questionnaire. Sleep Med 2012;13(2):172–7.

45. Cobb S, Jones JM. Social support, support groups and marital relationships. In: Duck S, editor. Personal relationships, vol. 5. London: Academic; 1984. p. 47–66.

46. Fotheringham MJ, Sawyer MG. Adherence to recommended medical regimens in childhood and adolescence. J Paediatr Child Health 1995;31(2): 72–8.

47. Weaver TE, Grunstein RR. Adherence to continuous positive airway pressure therapy: the challenge to effective treatment. Proc Am Thorac Soc 2008;5(2):173–8.

48. Strunk RC, Bender B, Young DA, et al. Predictors of protocol adherence in a pediatric asthma clinical trial. J Allergy Clin Immunol 2002;110(4): 596–602.

49. Smith BA, Shuchman M. Problem of nonadherence in chronically ill adolescents: strategies for assessment and intervention. Curr Opin Pediatr 2005; 17(5):613–8.

50. Khan M, Song X, Williams K, et al. Evaluating adherence to medication in children and adolescents with HIV. Arch Dis Child 2009;94(12): 970–3.

51. Chihara Y, Tsuboi T, Hitomi T, et al. Flexible positive airway pressure improves treatment adherence compared with auto-adjusting PAP. Sleep 2013; 36(2):229–36.

52. Bakker J, Campbell A, Neill A. Randomized controlled trial comparing flexible and continuous positive airway pressure delivery: effects on compliance, objective and subjective sleepiness and vigilance. Sleep 2010;33(4):523–9.

53. Chigier E. Compliance in adolescents with epilepsy or diabetes. J Adolesc Health 1992;13(5):375–9.

54. Orrell-Valente JK, Jarlsberg LG, Hill LG, et al. At what age do children start taking daily asthma medicines on their own? Pediatrics 2008;122(6): e1186–92.

55. Prashad PS, Marcus CL, Maggs J, et al. Investigating reasons for CPAP adherence in adolescents: a qualitative approach. J Clin Sleep Med 2013;9(12):1303–13.

56. Monaghan M, Horn I, Alvarez V, et al. Authoritative parenting, parenting stress, and self-care in preadolescents with Type 1 diabetes. J Clin Psychol Med S 2012;19:255–61.

57. Kirk VG, O'Donnell AR. Continuous positive airway pressure for children: a discussion on how to maximize compliance. Sleep Med Rev 2006;10(2): 119–27.

58. DiMatteo MR, Giordani PJ, Lepper HS, et al. Patient adherence and medical treatment outcomes: a meta-analysis. Med Care 2002;40(9): 794–811.

59. The Children's Hospital of Philadelphia. CPAP education: non-invasive ventilation for infants and children. 2013. Available at: http://www.chop.edu/service/sleep-center/cpap-education/non-invasive-ventilation-for-infants-and-children.html. Accessed November 25, 2013.

60. Ramirez A, Khirani S, Aloui S, et al. Continuous positive airway pressure and noninvasive ventilation adherence in children. Sleep Med 2013;14(12):1290–4.

61. Constantinidis J, Knobber D, Steinhart H, et al. Fine-structural investigations of the effect of nCPAP-mask application on the nasal mucosa. Acta Otolaryngol 2000;120(3):432–7.

62. Qureshi A, Ballard RD. Obstructive sleep apnea. J Allergy Clin Immunol 2003;112(4):643–51 [quiz: 652].

63. Waters KA, Everett FM, Bruderer JW, et al. Obstructive sleep apnea: the use of nasal CPAP in 80 children. Am J Respir Crit Care Med 1995; 152(2):780–5.

Myofunctional Therapy
A Novel Treatment of Pediatric Sleep-Disordered Breathing

Joy L. Moeller, BS, RDH[a],*,
Licia Coceani Paskay, MS, CCC-SLP[a],
Michael L. Gelb, DDS, MS[b]

KEYWORDS

• Myofunctional • Sleep • Breathing • Nasal • Tongue • Posture • Neuroplasticity • Assessment

KEY POINTS

- Orofacial myofunctional therapy (OMT) is a noninvasive option for the treatment of sleep-disordered breathing (SDB) in children.
- OMT has the potential to become an important alternative to other available nonsurgical treatment modalities.
- Early identification and correction of mouth breathing are recommended as early as the first year of life.
- Removing the tonsils and adenoids does not always change the breathing pattern from oral to nasal, if the habit of mouth breathing has not been corrected.
- Myofunctional therapists use a variety of supportive techniques to promote self-awareness and positive habits and to prevent the dysfunctions that characterize pediatric SDB.

INTRODUCTION

Orofacial myofunctional therapy (OMT) is defined as the treatment of dysfunctions of the muscles of the face and mouth, with the purpose of correcting orofacial functions, such as chewing and swallowing, and promoting nasal breathing. OMT has been used for many years to repattern and change the function of the oral and facial muscles and to eliminate oral habits, such as prolonged thumb-sucking and nail biting, tongue thrusting, open mouth at rest posture, incorrect mastication, and poor oral rest postures of the tongue and lips.[1] Physicians, dentists, and orthodontists have also used myofunctional therapy as an adjunctive noninvasive treatment of temporomandibular joint disorders (TMJD).

In the last few years[2,3] myofunctional therapy has also been proposed as a potentially important component of the multidisciplinary treatment of obstructive sleep apnea (OSA). The use of OMT as a noninvasive option for the treatment of sleep-disordered breathing (SDB) in children in particular represents a new and novel application of this well-established therapeutic approach and has the potential to become an important alternative to other available nonsurgical treatment modalities, such as positive airway pressure and

Disclosures: Paid lecturer for the Academy of Orofacial Myofunctional Therapy (AOMT), personally related to the AOMT Managing Director a main shareholder, Marc Moeller; Vice-president of the Academy of the 501(c)3 Academy of Applied Myofunctional Sciences (AAMS) (J.L. Moeller); Licia Coceani Paskay is a paid lecturer for the AOMT and President of the 501(c)3 AAMS (L.C. Paskay); No conflicts of interest (M.L. Gelb).
[a] Academy of Orofacial Myofunctional Therapy (AOMT), 910 Via de la Paz #106, Pacific Palisades, CA 90272, USA; [b] Department of Oral Medicine and Pathology, Tufts University School of Dental Medicine, NYU, 635 Madison Avenue, 19th Floor B/W: 59th & 60th Street, New York, NY 10022, USA
* Corresponding author.
E-mail address: joyleamoeller@aol.com

oral appliances. This article outlines the development and clinical application of OMT, discusses the rationale for its application to SDB, and presents evidence supporting this treatment as it relates to prevention, assessment, and treatment of pediatric SDB.

HISTORY OF OMT

The history of myofunctional therapy in the United States goes back to the early 1900s and parallels orthodontic treatment.[4] In the 1950s to 1960s, Walter Straub,[5,6] an orthodontist, wrote numerous articles on malfunctions of the tongue and abnormal swallowing habits and their relationship to orthodontics and speech. He thought a major cause of oral problems was bottle-feeding. Inspired by the work of Walter Straub, Roy Langer, Marvin Hanson, and Richard Barrett in the 1970s and 1980s, Daniel Garliner[7,8] was the first to recommend a therapeutic routine for nighttime sleeping consisting of keeping the lips together and the tongue up on the palate. Subsequently, 2 speech pathologists from Brazil, Irene Marchesan and Ester Bianchini, studied with Daniel Garliner in the 1980s and went back to Brazil, where they created a university program for speech pathologists centered on treating orofacial myofunctional disorders. Today, there are over 30 universities with PhD programs in myofunctional therapy and many programs that focus on sleep disorders and myofunctional therapy.

RATIONALE: DEVELOPMENT OF THE UPPER AIRWAY

As man evolved to an upright posture, the larynx descended, the forebrain grew, and the facial framework retreated, as the nasal airway became diminished in size and function. This evolution is one reason humans do not have the olfactory ability of other mammals. As the cranial base angle flexed, the maxilla was compressed and the paranasal sinus size was reduced, creating millions of sinus sufferers as well as other facial changes.

The flattened maxilla and longer face is a relatively recent phenomenon seen in humans, differentiating man from primates. The decrease in nose volume associated with cranial base flexing may have increased high upper airway resistance and increased the potential for collapse further down in the oropharynx. Man was no longer an obligate nose breather, and with increased demands, mouth breathing was born. This trend of mouth breathing, downward migration of the tongue base and descent of the hyoid, is associated with retrognathic changes in mandibular posture. The increase in mouth breathing is associated with less time spent with tongue to the palate, and therefore, with narrowing of the maxilla and an increased facial height. This downward and backward rotation of the maxilla and mandible is a powerful predictor of SDB as well as TMJD and malocclusion. A variety of researchers, clinicians, and anthropologists have identified an underdeveloped maxilla as being the root cause of malocclusion and naso-oropharyngeal constriction. Early identification of mouth breathing is therefore recommended as early as the first year of life.

Although the primary function of the genioglossus muscle is to protect the patency of the upper airway, an improper oral resting posture of the tongue will have a negative influence on the development of the oral cavity and the airway.[9] The anatomy of the upper airway in turn guides the growth and development of the nasomaxillary complex, mandible, temporomandibular joint, and ultimately, the occlusion of the teeth; thus, malocclusion and facial dysmorphism may be the result of compensation for a narrowed airway (**Fig. 1**).

Genioglossus Muscle Stabilizing the Airway

There are several etiologic factors that have been linked in varying degrees to the development of SDB in children, which have implications for the potential utility of OMT as a therapeutic intervention; these implications include feeding methods, oral habits, craniofacial abnormalities, hypertrophic tonsils and adenoids, chronic mouth breathing sleep position, and restricted frenum. For example, bottle-feeding has been shown to be a major contributing factor to an anterior open bite in the primary dentition,[10] whereas overuse of spouted ("sippy") cups may also contribute to a low tongue-rest posture, thereby leading to a narrow high palate. Oral habits such as the habitual use of a thumb or pacifier may also lead to a low tongue rest posture and OMD. It has been noted that the frequency, intensity, and duration of oral habits and mouth-soothing devices may lead to OMDs. When the thumb or another object is in the mouth often and/or for a prolonged period of time, as a self-soothing strategy for example, it applies pressure against the palate, and the tongue may develop a low rest posture. Also, incorrect pressure exerted on the jaws may lead to airway problems and a TMJD. Other oral habits such as finger-sucking, nail biting, lip biting or licking, and tongue sucking may develop in infancy and persist into adulthood, leading to malocclusion.[11]

Activity of the Genioglossus: Stabilizes and enlarges the portion of the upper airway that is most vulnerable to collapse (as in Sleep Disorders)

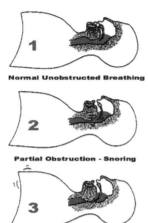

Normal Unobstructed Breathing

Partial Obstruction - Snoring

Complete Obstruction - OSA

Fig. 1. Genioglossus Muscle Stabilizing the Airways. (*From* Mathur R, Mortimore IL, Jan MA, et al. Effect of breathing, pressure and posture on palatoglossal and genioglossal tone. Clin Sci 1995;89:441–45; with permission.)

Mouth breathing or an open mouth at rest may be one cause of OMDs. If the mouth is open, the tongue usually rests down and forward. This position may cause an abnormal growth pattern, which may lead to a forward head and neck posture, malocclusion, and SDB.[12] Mouth breathing also involves lack of lip closure, which is necessary for jaw stability and to create the intraoral negative pressure necessary to hold the tongue in place. Moreover, in mouth breathing there is a lack of tongue-to-palate contact, necessary to create the "suction-cup" effect that holds the tongue in place and prevents it from falling into the pharynx.

Hypertrophic tonsils and adenoids may also lead to OMD and SDB. If the palatine tonsils are hypertrophic, the tongue is prevented from swallowing properly, forcing the tongue to come forward during the swallow and to rest forward and down. However, removing the tonsils and adenoids does not always change the breathing pattern from oral to nasal, especially in the long-term. A myofunctional therapist may be needed to assist the child in retraining the function of the tongue, in breathing, chewing, and swallowing, and to eliminate maladaptive oral habits. Finally, restricted lingual or labial frena may cause an OMD[13]; if the tongue is not able to create a vacuum seal on the palate, then a high and narrow palate may result, which is considered to be a risk factor for OSA (**Fig. 2**).[14]

Several studies support an empiric basis for myofunctional therapy in the treatment of SDB in adults. In an often-referenced study, Guimarães and colleagues[15] reported not only reduced symptoms of sleep apnea but also objective evidence of decreased disease severity. The study reports that the apnea/hypopnea index (AHI) was reduced by 39% in those patients, after 3 months of myofunctional therapy. More recently, a series of studies on the application of myofunctional therapy of SDB in children from Stanford University showed that the addition of myofunctional therapy to adenotonsillectomy or palatal expansion reduced the risk of reoccurrence of SDB. A retrospective investigation by Guilleminault and colleagues[3] evaluated the application of myofunctional therapy along with adenotonsillectomy and orthodontic treatment. In patients who received myofunctional therapy, the AHI and the oxygen desaturation were normalized, whereas most subjects who did not receive myofunctional therapy experienced a relapse in both the AHI and the mean minimum oxygen saturation. The authors conclude that the absence of myofascial (myofunctional) treatment is associated with an increased risk of SDB recurrence.

Although studies that show a specific effect of myofunctional therapy on children's sleep is relatively small, research supporting that OMT indeed normalizes the basic orofacial functions involved in SDB[16,17] is more robust. For example, Izu and colleagues[18] found that oral breathers were more likely to have snoring and OSAs and suffer from adenotonsillitis and otological symptoms. Cunha and colleagues[19] found that breathing abnormalities in children not only alter sleep but affect chewing and food intake. Normalizing orofacial functions in children also requires time. Marson and colleagues[20] demonstrated the effectiveness of an OMT program to normalize nasal breathing with peak results at 12 weeks, whereas Gallo and Campiotto,[21]

Tongue mobility (best result = 0 e worst result = 14). Final result =

	Successful	Partially successful	Unsuccessful
Protrude and retract	(0)	(1)	(2)
Touch the upper lip with the apex	(0)	(1)	(2)
Touch the right commissura labiorum	(0)	(1)	(2)
Touch the left commissura labiorum	(0)	(1)	(2)
Touch U&L molars	(0)	(1)	(2)
Apex vibration	(0)	(1)	(2)
Sucking against the palate	(0)	(1)	(2)

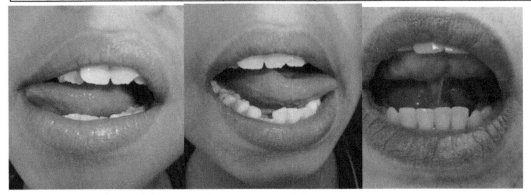

Fig. 2. Determining the need for a Lingual Frenectomy: Mobility Test.

using a similar protocol, found nasal breathing was normalized after about 10 sessions.

CLINICAL ASSESSMENT

Every health professional who works with patients with sleep disorders has different tools available for assessment, based on their needs, scope of practice, and preferences. Myofunctional therapists, as a multidisciplinary group of professionals, use various tools and practices, which often overlap but retain some individual characteristics depending on the background of the therapist. Moreover, myofunctional therapists are trained to identify other underlying orofacial dysfunctions that are affected or are a contributing factor in sleep disorders.

As part of the standard evaluation, the orofacial myofunctional therapist takes a thorough medical and developmental history, with an emphasis on SDB risk factors. Important components of the assessment include identification of oral habits that interfere with a proper oral rest posture, recognition of the incorrect rest position of the tongue, determination of incorrect swallow, labial and lingual frenum restriction and inadequate lip seal, and evaluation of functional head and neck posture (after age 3–4 years) (**Figs. 3–14**).

Fig. 3. Thumb habit.

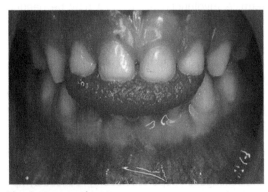

Fig. 4. Tongue thrust.

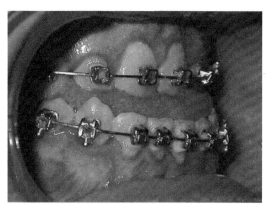

Fig. 5. Tongue rest position.

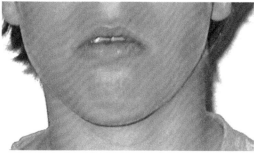

Fig. 8. Open lips at rest: may be flacid, swollen or cracked.

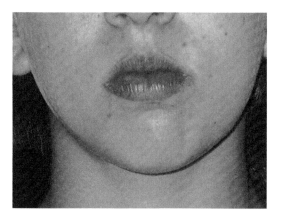

Fig. 6. Over-developed mentalis muscle.

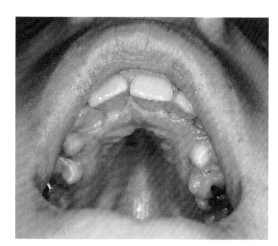

Fig. 9. High narrow palate.

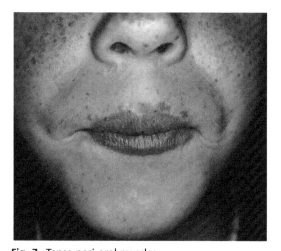

Fig. 7. Tense peri-oral muscles.

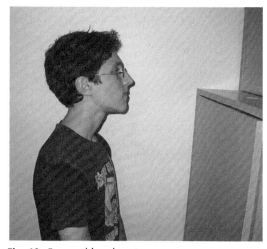

Fig. 10. Forward head posture.

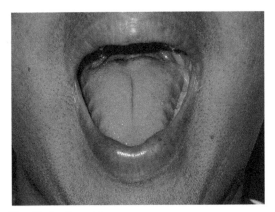

Fig. 11. Scalloped tongue.

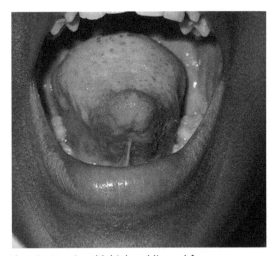

Fig. 13. Restricted labial and lingual frena.

Treatment

Treatment consists of habit elimination and behavior modification, jaw stabilization exercises, repatterning the oral facial muscles and changing their function for optimal nasal breathing, oral rest position, chewing, and swallowing. There are 4 basic components to the treatment:

1. Restoring Proper Rest Oral Posture

   The first step is to educate the patient about problematic oral habits they may have and how to modify or eliminate the behavior, in terms of reduced frequency, duration, and the intensity of the habit. Myofunctional therapists use a variety of supportive techniques to allow the patient to first understand the damage being done and then to solicit a commitment to change, even in young children. Then, the patient is supported with rewards and positive reinforcement from both the family and the therapist. Therapists then will introduce diaphragmatic breathing and create a lip seal (in the absence of airway blockages or allergies), so that the lips are closed during the night. Therapy then continues with training the blade of the tongue to go to the "spot," which is located posterior to the first rugae or ridge posterior to the maxillary central incisors on the palate. This therapy will also help to substitute the thumb with the tongue if necessary.

2. Repatterning of Facial Muscles

   Next, the therapist will work with a sequential set of exercises to activate and then repattern the oral facial muscles. Therapists work with the muscles of mastication, which support the mandible and which

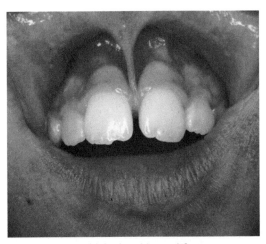

Fig. 12. Restricted labial and lingual frena.

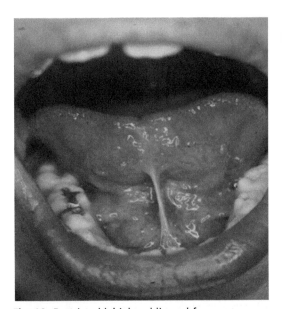

Fig. 14. Restricted labial and lingual frena.

aid the proper position of the genioglossus at night. Then, additional training addresses the orbicularis oris as well as the intrinsic and extrinsic tongue muscles, the buccinators, and the perioral muscles.

3. Teaching Proper Chewing and Swallowing

Next, proper chewing and swallowing is gradually introduced. Proper oral posture is reinforced even during sleep, with subconscious auto-suggestion and biofeedback. Success is evaluated using the Mallampati score, the grade of tongue scalloping, relaxation, or activation of the perioral muscles, as well as attaining a lip seal and palatal tongue rest position during both the day and the night.

4. Functional posture training

Myofunctional therapists are trained to promote a functional head position during sleep, to avoid the jaw being in close proximity to the chest because this position may contribute to SDB. Also, OMTs instruct patients to hold an upright head and neck posture, especially during the swallowing process.

If myofunctional therapists suspect that the "tongue-tie" (or lip-tie) is contributing to a child's SDB, they will evaluate both the labial and the lingual frena, usually after a few weeks of exercises to ensure that full range of motion of the tongue and lips is possible. If the restriction remains, the patient is referred to a physician or dentist who is comfortable doing the surgery. After the release, the patient must immediately do exercises to assure proper function of the tongue. Otherwise, more revisions may be required.

The key to successful treatment is to establish a rapport with the pediatric patient and the caregiver and to motivate and monitor the outcome on a weekly basis for several months and then gradually reduce the frequency of appointments to once a month. The therapist must also enlist the assistance of the parent or caregiver to become the "therapist" at home to assure a successful result.

Because myofunctional therapy relies on active patient participation, OMTs use several techniques that are based on the 10 principles of neuroplasticity.[22] Neuroplasticity means the ability of the brain to change, following physiologic or pathologic input, generating an adaptive response. These principles include the following.

Use it or lose it

In general, because muscle function requires energy, if the muscles are not properly used, the brain stops or reduces nourishing those muscles and hypotonia may follow. Two studies[23] indicated that loss of prolonged sensory input translates to a reduction of the somatocortical representation, such as in children with a habitual open mouth during the day and at night.

Use it and improve it

Myofunctional therapy revolves around the principle of improving a function through repetition, metacognition, and awareness. For example, the tongue is repositioned and trained to contact the palate comfortably, thus providing the natural negative pressure (suction) that keeps the tongue, and especially the genioglossus, in the proper position during sleep.[15,24]

Plasticity is experience specific

This principle suggests that the success of some therapy protocols for sleep disorders[15] relies on targeting the very muscles that are hypofunctioning at night, such as the soft palate, tongue, and pharyngeal walls.

Repetition matters

"Practice" improves performance by creating, maintaining, and expanding new neural areas corresponding to the new behavior. In myofunctional therapy repetition is paramount so that a new behavior, such as the tongue position or lips closure, is rehearsed every day and every evening until the new habit is formed.

Intensity matters

Ideally, patients should practice neuromuscular exercises every day; otherwise, the intensity of the neuromuscular change does not generalize to the night hours.

Time matters

According to Fisher and Sullivan,[16,25] the training modality that is most effective is protracted and continuous, as opposed to brief and intermittent. Therefore, patients may need to be kept in therapy or follow-up mode for a prolonged period of time (usually 1 year, but 2 years is better for habituation).

Salience matters

The need to motivate the patient by increasing the saliency or importance of therapy is a central element, because the higher the motivation and understanding of the reason some exercises need to be performed daily, the more likely the patient will perform the exercises prescribed.

Age matters

Children are in the best condition to transform sensory-motor inputs into correct functions and

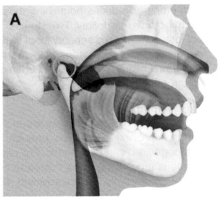 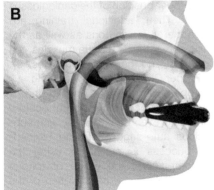

Fig. 15. (A) and (B) Airway Centric ™ Philosophy.

make them a life-long habit. In children, not only is neuroplasticity at its best but also muscles and soft tissues drive the development of bones through principles of the functional matrix and epigenetic influences.[17,26]

Transference

The transference principle supports the co-occurrence of multiple functions when an overlapping one has been established.[27] When the patient breathes well through the nose, other functions can now easily take place even if they were hampered before, such as tongue repositioning or lip seal.

Interference

When a patient learns a new behavior (such as nasal breathing), the old behavior (such as oral breathing) has the ability to interfere neurologically with the establishment of the new one. It is only by continuous repetition of the new behavior and suppression of the old one that plasticity occurs.

Because a transition from daily myofunctional retraining to nocturnal activities, when the brain is not directly engaged, requires a good degree of patience and perseverance, building motivation relies on the skills of the therapist. Motivation assists the development of habituation, which is a function of time (now, later, or in the future). In therapy, feedback must be used constantly, be it visual, auditory, or tactile. Therapy implies self-talk, but a visual reminder or touch stimulus may be needed as well.

Myofunctional therapy alone may be successful in treating mild-to-moderate SDB, but in many children with SDB, the best results are achieved with a combination of patient myofunctional retraining and other therapeutic options, such as adenotonsillectomy, oral appliances, or positive airway pressure (**Fig. 15**). Although more research is needed to document the effectiveness of OMT in

the treatment as well as the prevention of SDB in the pediatric population, the potential benefits of including a myofunctional therapist in a team approach should not be underestimated.

REFERENCES

1. Hanson ML. Orofacial myofunctional therapy: historical and philosophical considerations. Int J Orofacial Myology 1988;14(1):3–10.
2. Huang YS, Guilleminault C. Pediatric obstructive sleep apnea and the critical role of oral-facial growth: evidence. Front Neurol 2013;3:184. http://dx.doi.org/10.3389/fneur.2012.00184 (18).
3. Guilleminault C, Huang YS, Monteyrol PJ, et al. Critical role of myofascial reeducation in pediatric sleep-disordered breathing. Sleep Med 2013;14(6):518–25.
4. Levrini A, Favero L. The masters of functional orthodontics. Carol Stream (IL): Quintessence Publishing Co; 2003.
5. Straub WJ. Malfunction of the tongue. Part I. The abnormal swallowing habit: its causes, effects, and results in relation to orthodontic treatment and speech therapy. Am J Orthod 1960;46:404–24.
6. Straub WJ. Malfunction of the tongue. Part II. The abnormal swallowing habit: its causes, effects, and results in relation to orthodontic treatment and speech therapy. Am J Orthod 1961;47:596–617.
7. Garliner D. Myofunctional therapy in dental practice: abnormal swallowing habits: diagnosis-treatment. Brooklyn (NY): Bartel Dental Book Company, Inc; 1971.
8. Garliner D. Myofunctional therapy. Philadelphia: W. B. Saunders; 1976.
9. Mathur R, Mortimore IL, Jan MA, et al. Effect of breathing, pressure and posture on palatoglossal and genioglossal tone. Clin Sci 1995;89:441–5.
10. Romero CC, Scavone-Junior H, Garib DG, et al. Breastfeeding and non-nutritive sucking patterns related to the prevalence of anterior open bite in

primary dentition. J Appl Oral Sci 2011;19(2): 161–8.

11. Quashie-Williams R, daCosta OO, Isiekwe MC. Oral habits, prevalence and effects on occlusion of 4-15 year old school children in Lagos, Nigeria. Niger Postgrad Med J 2010;17(2):113–7.

12. Bonuck KA, Chervin RD, Cole TJ, et al. Prevalence and persistence of sleep disordered breathing symptoms in young children: a 6-year population-based cohort study. Sleep 2011;34(7):875–84.

13. Northcutt M. Overview the lingual frenum. J Clin Orthod 2009;18:557–65.

14. Kushida C, Efron B, Guilleminault C. A predictive morphometric model for the obstructive sleep apnea syndrome. Ann Intern Med 1997;127(8 Pt 1): 581–7.

15. Guimarães KC, Drager LF, Genta PR, et al. Effects of oropharyngeal exercises on patients with moderate obstructive sleep apnea syndrome. Am J Respir Crit Care Med 2009;179(10):962–6. http://dx.doi.org/10.1164/rccm.200806-981OC.

16. Silva LM, Aureliano FT, Motta AR. Speech therapy in the obstructive sleep apnea-hypopnea syndrome: case report. Rev. CEFAC 2007;9(4):490–6. http://dx.doi.org/10.1590/S1516-18462007000400009.

17. Landa PG, Suzuki HS. Sleep obstructive apnea-hypoapnea syndrome and the phonoaudiological focus: literature review. Rev. CEFAC 2009;11(3):507–15. http://dx.doi.org/10.1590/S1516-18462009000300020.

18. Izu SC, Itamoto CH, Pradella-Hallinan M, et al. Obstructive sleep apnea syndrome (OSAS) in mouth breathing children. Braz J Otorhinolaryngol 2010;76(5):552–6. http://dx.doi.org/10.1590/S1808-86942010000500003.

19. Cunha DA, da Silva GA, Motta ME, et al. Mouth breathing in children and its repercussions in the nutritional state. Rev CEFAC 2007;9(1):47–54. http://dx.doi.org/10.1590/S1516-18462007000100007.

20. Marson A, Tessitore A, Sakano E, et al. Effectiveness of speech and language therapy and brief intervention proposal in mouth breathers. Rev CEFAC 2012; 14(6):1153–66. http://dx.doi.org/10.1590/S1516-18462012005000054.

21. Gallo J, Campiotto AR. Myofunctional therapy in children with oral breathing. Rev CEFAC 2009; 11(Suppl 3):305–10. http://dx.doi.org/10.1590/S1516-18462009000700005.

22. Robbins J, Butler SG, Daniels SK, et al. Swallowing and dysphagia rehabilitation: translating principles of neural plasticity into clinically oriented evidence. J Speech Lang Hear Res 2008;51(1):S276–300. http://dx.doi.org/10.1044/1092-4388(2008/021).

23. Merzenich MM, Kaas JH, Wall JT, et al. Progression of change following median nerve section in the cortical representation of the hand in areas 3b and 1 in adult owl and squirrel monkeys. Neuroscience 1983;10:639–65.

24. Engelke W, Jung K, Knosel M. Intra-oral compartment pressures: a biofunctional model and experimental measurements under different conditions of posture. Clin Oral Investig 2011;15(2):165–76.

25. Fisher BE, Sullivan KJ. Activity-dependent factors affecting poststroke functional outcomes. Top Stroke Rehabil 2001;8(3):31–44.

26. Moss M. The functional matrix hypothesis revisited. 1. The role of mechanotransduction. Am J Orthod Dentofacial Orthop 1997;112(1):8–11.

27. Kleim JA, Jones TA. Principles of experience-dependent neural plasticity: implications for rehabilitation after brain damage. J Speech Lang Hear Res 2008;51(1):S225–39.

Setting Up a Child-Friendly Sleep Laboratory

Patrick Sorenson, MA, RPSGT[a], Judith A. Owens, MD, MPH[b],*

KEYWORDS

- Pediatric polysomnography • Family-centered approach • Electroencephalogram
- Electrooculogram (EOG) • Electromyogram • Safety • Functionality

KEY POINTS

- Environmental concerns include adequate spacial concerns for all family members and employees to provide a safe and functional facility in which to perform polygraphic testing on children.
- Personnel considerations specific to pediatric polysomnography that require specific training in pediatrics using a family-centered approach include schedulers, managerial, technical, and medical staff, but may also include emergency personnel, nursing personnel, social workers, transportation, translators, and security personnel.
- Considerations that contain specific concepts for those sleep laboratories performing pediatric polysomnographic evaluations include the data acquisition system, technological staffing and approaches, the sleep study request or order form, the reporting of findings, and the follow-up.
- The evaluation of polysomnograms in the pediatric population includes accepted scoring guidelines by personnel specifically trained to perform this task and are aware of the different facets found in pediatric sleep that may or may not conform to the accepted guidelines.

INTRODUCTION

There are many developmental, operational, and environmental aspects to consider when structuring a safe environment in which to perform procedures intended to assist in the diagnosis and treatment of sleep disorders in the pediatric population. This article will outline some of the basic current concepts that are important in establishing a consensus within either a new pediatric sleep medicine team, or in a well-established team looking for more guidance or information on how to improve services for children. This consensus building within the sleep laboratory team is necessary to function efficiently on all operational levels; basic concepts include but are not limited to challenges in the scheduling, performance,

scoring, and interpretation of diagnostic pediatric polysomnograms (PSG) and treatment studies (eg, positive airway pressure titration).

In those laboratories that are currently studying children, there is likely already an awareness of specific challenges that can lead to frustration and stress within the team, as well as those that impact on the quality of the sleep laboratory experience for children and their families. This article is geared both toward more and less experienced laboratories in regards to treating children (ie, laboratories that exclusively serve adults and older adolescents, mixed laboratories, and those that are solely pediatric-focused); however some presumptions have been made in regards to the reader having a basic level of knowledge about policies and procedures instrumental to operating a sleep

Conflict of Interest: None.
[a] Sleep Laboratory, Department of Sleep Medicine, Children's National Medical Center, 111 Michigan Avenue NW, Washington, DC 20010-2970, USA; [b] Children's National Medical Center, George Washington University School of Medicine and Health Sciences, 111 Michigan Avenue NW, Washington, DC 20010-2970, USA
* Corresponding author.
E-mail address: owensleep@gmail.com

laboratory. Finally, a detailed discussion of the interpretation of pediatric sleep studies, while vitally important, is beyond the scope of this article, as are special considerations in managing children on positive airway pressure treatment[1] (see article by Marcus and colleagues in this issue.)

In order for a laboratory to function optimally when working with the pediatric population, the team should consist of personnel specifically trained and experienced in working with children and families, from the point of initial contact throughout the entire process of conducting, scoring, and interpreting the study.[2] At all of the stages there are opportunities to incorporate a family-centered approach. It is especially important to recognize not only the differences between conducting polysomnography in adults and children, but also the variety of issues raised within different pediatric subpopulations; these include children across the developmental spectrum and with a variety of medical and psychiatric conditions. These considerations are particularly important, because in recent years more primarily adult sleep laboratories have been considering expanding services to the pediatric population; this is at least, in part, a means of off-setting the decline in in-laboratory adult studies due to the transition to in-home portable monitoring. Thus, these laboratories may not be adequately equipped to handle children and families. On the other hand, adequate numbers of pediatric laboratories to handle the numbers of children needing sleep studies do not yet exist. Thus, a compromise that ensures that all sleep laboratories purporting to study children meet minimum standards is imperative.

SETTING UP A CHILD-FRIENDLY SLEEP LABORATORY

In order to comprehensively cover the fundamental aspects necessary to establish and maintain a safe and child-friendly sleep laboratory, it will be necessary to provide a discussion of such issues as pediatric-specific environmental and safety considerations, personnel requirements, basic procedural guidelines, management strategies, and some specific technical/equipment aspects.

Environmental Considerations

Environmental concerns that will need to be addressed for the successful pediatric sleep laboratory include functional as well as safety aspects as follows, with some overlap between the two:

- The proper planning of the laboratory environment will include bedrooms that have adequate space for several reasons. First, the caregiver, usually the parent, should remain in the laboratory for the duration of the study for the comfort of the child as well as his or her safety. Moreover, in most states, children less 18 years old cannot give consent to medical procedures unless they are an emancipated minor, and thus must be accompanied by an adult. Therefore, a separate and comfortable bed for caregivers is a necessity.
- Another universally recognized requirement for any sleep laboratory environment is that the bedroom size must be adequate for technologists and emergency personnel to function properly. However, in the pediatric population additional personnel who may be involved in providing adequate safety and comfort measures include nurses, social workers, transportation personnel, translators, and even security personnel. The more complex the medical, developmental, and familial situation of the child who is being seen in the laboratory, the more likely these personnel will be needed and will need to be readily available during the duration of patient's visit.
- In addition to providing adequate space, the bedrooms should have soundproofing adequate to minimize sound from carrying into other areas of the laboratory, particularly if the laboratory serves both adults and children. The soundproofing process may add significantly to construction costs but should be considered a critical aspect of the planning of any sleep laboratory evaluating pediatric patients.
- Whether the physical location of the sleep medicine clinic and the sleep laboratory are to be separate or one in the same, decisions about optimal structure and workflow are important considerations. In regards to these considerations, there may be advantages to dual use of the sleep laboratory space for PSG testing by night and clinical evaluation (ie, sleep clinic) by day. These include improved cost: benefit ratios due to sharing of administrative personnel and repurposing unused space into revenue-generating space during the day, and promotion of a more family-centered approach by providing patients and caregivers with an increased comfort level with the physical location and arrangement. Rooms that double as both a clinic and polysomnographic laboratory space can be efficiently converted for either use with prefabricated wall systems (eg,

convertible Murphy bed and examination table) (**Fig. 1**).

Safety Considerations

In regards to safety, standard items in a pediatric sleep facility environment should include

- Exogenous oxygen, air, and suctioning capabilities
- A crash cart with a range of supplies for patients of any age, including infant populations if necessary
- Bedside resuscitation equipment such as resuscitation equipment and masks
- Plastic safety covers for unused outlets
- Safe and approved furniture including bedding with features such as railings with no-pinch moving parts and seizure pads
- A safe, locked area in which to store hazardous substances used in sleep laboratories such as bleach, cleansers, and collodion

Additional important safety considerations may include

- Elimination of hazardous pull cords used for blinds or similar equipment
- Active and/or passive prevention of patient unfettered access to the monitoring equipment and sensors
- Child-friendly lighting sources that cannot be tipped or easily broken
- The ability to independently alter the temperature of testing rooms (eg, this can help prevent sweat artifact known to adversely affect the recording or provide an appropriate sleep environment for infants)

Finally, from a more practical standpoint, there are additional modifications to consider in order to enhance safety and functionality:

- Use of moisture-resistant and easy-to-clean mattresses and pillow covers
- Adjustable intensity of ambient lighting (eg, dimmer switch)
- Blinds and shading that can eliminate outside light and reduce sound contamination
- Easily accessible and ubiquitous alcohol-based hand cleansers

Personnel and Staff

Any diagnostic or treatment procedure involving children should be conducted by medical personnel who are specifically trained to address behavioral and physiologic aspects of disordered sleep in children. A sleep technologist is also often working with children during a time of day when the child's behavior is at its most dysregulated, with caregivers whose patience may be stretched thin and in an environment that is unfamiliar and may be intimidating for families. In this regard, it is strongly suggested that only those technologists who want to work with children and who understand the added difficulties in studying this population be given the responsibility of working with them. A seasoned pediatric technologist will be able to assess each patient and use appropriate sensors and techniques to obtain an optimal sleep study. During the hiring and initial training process, it is critical for the success of the new technologist to be well versed in all of the specific policies and procedures of the laboratory. This will be time well spent in that a knowledgeable technologist can produce and troubleshoot pediatric recordings to minimize poor or missing data and can function independently. A

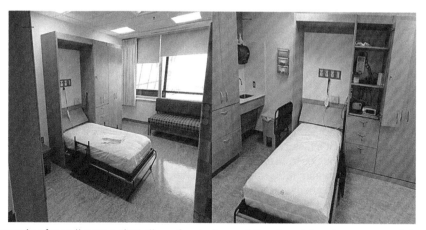

Fig. 1. An example of a wall system that allows for dual use of the sleep laboratory space and daytime clinical evaluation of children.

good technologist takes individualized care of each patient and family, and this will clearly show in the quality of the PSG.

The sleep laboratory manager provides an important interface between the administrative and technical staff, the medical director, and other personnel tangentially associated with the laboratory. Managerial personnel assure the proper day-to-day operations of the laboratory, are responsible for developing and adhering to evidence-based policies and procedures of the laboratory specific to the pediatric population, and provide oversight of education and training of both the scheduling and technical staff. In addition, technical oversight is frequently necessary to provide advice or suggestions to achieve the goal of artifact-free recordings.

POLICIES AND PROCEDURES

Whether a mixed (ie, adult and child, pediatric sleep clinic and laboratory) or dedicated space, the team should have child-specific policies and procedures in place to ensure that operations (eg, scheduling, charting, and dissemination of information) are seamless and efficient; organized and regular interface with laboratory and administrative and managerial personnel should be clearly delineated for smooth operations. Key aspects of child- and family-friendly policies include referral procedures and scheduling.

Referral Procedures

The request for a sleep study on a pediatric patient should include information that may not be typically requested for sleep studies in adult populations. This information is critical to ensuring the safety of the child in the laboratory, as well as to accurate production and interpretation of PSG data and thus to the integrity and value of the results. Inappropriate scheduling and inadequate staffing, difficulties in the set-up procedure, and misinterpretation of the data collected are all potential consequences associated with inadequate or inaccurate patient information accompanying the PSG request.

In addition to demographic information and the reason(s) for which the study is being requested, all pediatric referrals should be accompanied by a pertinent details of the patient's history and physical examination, as well as findings from any previous sleep or electroencephalogram (EEG) studies. The history and physical examination findings should at minimum include details regarding the child's upper airway (including the types and dates of prior surgeries [eg, adenotonsillectomy], tonsillar size, Mallampati score, presence of craniofacial abnormalities including retrognathia and micrognathia), any history of cardiovascular or respiratory disease, and presence of symptoms of (eg, snoring or observed apneic pauses) and risk factors for sleep disordered breathing (eg, positive family history, obesity, or allergic rhinitis). Additional critical pieces of information that should be requested include the presence of comorbid syndromes or medical conditions, current medications, developmental considerations (eg, global developmental delay or intellectual disability), and any known behavioral issues (eg, autism spectrum disorder).

The referral form should also clearly define any special orders, including Positive Airway Pressure (PAP) titration (initial or repeat), administration of exogenous O_2, or additional EEG leads to either rule out abnormal epileptiform central nervous system (CNS) activity or more comprehensively evaluate the CNS, as is sometimes critical for infants. Other separate orders may include a multiple sleep latency test (MSLT) or a pH study to help rule out gastroesophageal reflux (GER).

Scheduling

Scheduling concerns specific to the pediatric population require heightened organizational skills, a knowledge base specific to the special needs of children and their families, an in-depth knowledge of the requirements of third party payers, and lots of patience. Once the request for a pediatric sleep study is reviewed by the responsible physician or his or her designate, decisions as to how to schedule the study may be influenced by the acuity of the patient, the needs of the family and child, the requests of the referring health care provider, and the specific policies of the laboratory in regards to scheduling children. Considerations such as work, school, and family schedules often need to be balanced with availability of testing rooms and staff. Similar to any aspect of conducting pediatric sleep studies, scheduling requires a family-centered approach and a respectful family–professional partnership that honors the strengths, cultures, traditions, and expertise that everyone brings to the interaction.[3] For example, the almost universal requirement that only one caregiver accompany the child under 18 years of age for the duration of the study can yield significant consequences (eg, for a single parent with other siblings in the home). Although some laboratories may allow two or perhaps more caregivers to remain during the set up procedure, once the study is begun, the room can be occupied by only the 1 caregiver and the patient to maintain a controlled environment during the study. Thus, these policies should be made clear during scheduling, to allow ample time for planning alternative childcare and transportation arrangements and to minimize misunderstandings. In addition, the encouragement of family-to-family or peer support can often provide the needed solutions. These successes should be celebrated with the caregivers for their use of problem-solving skills and for the positive effect on future interactions with the sleep laboratory staff and subsequent medical professionals.

Finally, scheduling pediatric patients for sleep studies including those that are medically complicated, requires the timely notification of staff for special requirements, including cribs for younger children, a Hoyer Lift for paraplegic or quadriplegic patients, and any special nutritional needs (eg, overnight continuous gastrostomy tube feeds). In this regard, a competent scheduler is often considered the nerve center for the laboratory and as such is invaluable to the smooth operations of the pediatric sleep laboratory. The scheduler must often deal with issues that may compound the efforts needed to get a child appropriately studied, including last-minute cancellations or patients who fail to show for appointments. Scheduling sleep studies for pediatric patients requires patience, tact and, at times, a healthy sense of humor.

TECHNICAL CONSIDERATIONS

Technical considerations for pediatric polysomnography include the use of specialized age-appropriate equipment and appropriate attachment to patients and accurate interface with data acquisition systems also designed with the younger populations in mind. There will be different technical approaches to the sleep study production not necessarily based on chronological age but also the developmental age of the patient.

Careful consideration should be given to these technical aspects of the testing environment, including use of a data collection system that can accurately collect and portray the idiosyncrasies of pediatric sleep and age-appropriate sensors and materials. These data acquisition considerations include but are not limited to

- Multiple-channel capacity, including expanded EEG data
- Appropriate filtering, remontaging and re-referencing capability
- Adequate shielding of cables to reduce or eliminate stray currents from infiltrating the system and obscuring the data, as the use of a notch (60 Hz) filter on EEG data may be inappropriate in the pediatric population
- Ease of appropriate handling of sometimes extended periods of artifactual data

- The ability to adjust the window (paper speed) to visualize the data at any desired speed; since infants and toddlers often breathe rapidly, visualizing respiratory data at 120 seconds/page would be inappropriate, and 60 to 90 seconds/page may be more advantageous
- The ability to record and report elevated heart rates
- A clear and adjustable video system positioned appropriately above the bed at an angle where the patient's face is clearly and easily visible
- An audio system positioned as close to the patient's head as possible to capture even very soft snoring or other breathing sounds

In addition, diagnostic systems should include an easily customizable PSG report template specific to children, with the ability to generate separate reports for special populations, such as infants.

The pediatric sleep laboratory should be well stocked with different age-appropriate sensors either developed specifically for children or deemed appropriate for use in even very young children. Although there are many different sensors available, those with a good track record for providing accurate data in pediatric populations are usually well known and easily available commercially. Sensors made specifically for children include oxygen saturation (SpO_2) monitors and probes, snore sensors such as a microphone or vibration sensor, size-specific cannulas for measuring end-tidal CO_2 ($EtCO_2$) or ionization sensors for monitoring transcutaneous CO_2 (tCO_2), airflow sensors designed to ideally remain on even in a moist environment, and a respiratory inductive plethysmograph effort belt system that can provide a summation channel.

SUMMARY

Although there are many aspects to consider when studying the sleep of children, there are basic concepts that should be seriously considered when this age group is accepted into the sleep laboratory. The difficulties associated with studying this age group can certainly be reduced with an increase awareness of the inherent differences seen in this population as compared to adult polysomnography. These differences are multifaceted and are seen in areas such as the environment, safety, functionality, and coherent evidence-based policies. Although these areas of potential difficulties can be found in any aspect pediatric medicine, including polysomnography, there are also many opportunities for success. When performed optimally, pediatric polysomnography can be a rich and rewarding experience for the sleep laboratory team, patients, and families.

REFERENCES

1. Marcus CL, Beck SE, Traylor J, et al. Randomized, double-blind clinical trial of two different modes of positive airway pressure therapy on adherence and efficacy in children. J Clin Sleep Med 2012;8(1):37–42.

2. National Center for Family-Centered Care. Family-centered care for children with special health care needs. Bethesda (MD): Association for the Care of Children's Health; 1989.

3. Berry R, Brooks R, Gamaldo C, et al. The AASM manual for the scoring of sleep and associated events – rules, terminology and technical specifications V. 2.0. American Academy of Sleep Medicine; 2012.

Controversies in Behavioral Treatment of Sleep Problems in Young Children

Jocelyn H. Thomas, PhD[a], Melisa Moore, PhD[a],
Jodi A. Mindell, PhD[a,b],*

KEYWORDS

- Sleep • Young children • Behavioral intervention • Age • Sleep aids • Pharmacologic agents
- Child and family outcomes

KEY POINTS

- Behavioral interventions to treat sleep problems in young children are efficacious and should be tailored to meet the needs of the individual child and family.
- Evidence suggests that treatment strategies can be initiated after 3 to 4 months of age and may include a sleep aid as a noncritical component.
- Pharmacologic agents are not likely to be effective as the sole intervention, and behavioral strategies should be used as the primary treatment procedure.
- Behavioral treatments have not been found to have iatrogenic effects on the child, parent, or parent-child relationship.

Sleep problems are a common parent complaint, with estimates that approximately 30% of children experience some difficulty sleeping.[1,2] Trouble falling asleep and waking during the night are the most prevalent concerns for young children and occur in 20% to 30% of infants, toddlers, and preschool-aged children.[3,4] In addition, longitudinal studies have shown that sleep difficulties may persist for months to years and can become a chronic problem. For example, a longitudinal study of 359 mother/child pairs found that 21% of children with sleep problems in infancy, compared with 6% of those without, had sleep problems in the third year of life.[5] Furthermore, sleep problems can have a negative impact on mood, behavior, academic achievement, learning, and memory consolidation.[6,7] Untreated sleep problems are also a public health concern as insufficient and inappropriately timed sleep has been linked to an increased risk of obesity and a considerable estimated economic burden.[8,9]

Treatment options and the implementation of intervention procedures may seem confusing and overwhelming to parents (especially to those who are sleep deprived). Practitioners also often look for guidance. This article seeks to address some of the most frequent controversial issues and common questions related to the implementation of behavioral interventions in young children, including (1) which behavioral techniques have the most empiric support, (2) what is the best age to begin to implement these strategies, (3) should sleep aids or transitional objects be used, (4) what is the role of pharmacologic agents as an adjunct to behavioral interventions, and finally (5) what are the potential negative consequences

a Sleep Center, Division of Pulmonary Medicine, Children's Hospital of Philadelphia, Civic Center Boulevard, Philadelphia, PA 19104, USA; b Department of Psychology, Saint Joseph's University, City Avenue, Philadelphia, PA 19131, USA
* Corresponding author. Department of Psychology, Saint Joseph's University, Philadelphia, PA 19131.
E-mail address: jmindell@sju.edu

Sleep Med Clin 9 (2014) 251–259
http://dx.doi.org/10.1016/j.jsmc.2014.02.004
1556-407X/14/$ – see front matter © 2014 Elsevier Inc. All rights reserved.

of implementing behavioral interventions on the child, parent, and the child-parent relationship.

WHICH TECHNIQUE IS BEST FOR INFANT AND TODDLER SLEEP DISTURBANCES?

A variety of behavioral treatment methods have been shown to be efficacious in the treatment of sleep problems in young children and are both widely recommended in clinical practice and used by parents with or without professional guidance.[3] However, parents as well as practitioners may be overwhelmed with the variety of behavioral approaches and have difficulty choosing which intervention to implement.

Most behavioral strategies are based on the premise that difficulties falling asleep and frequent awakenings throughout the night are related to parental involvement at the time of sleep onset. If parents habitually assist their child in falling asleep at bedtime, the child may not be given the opportunity to develop the self-regulatory skills necessary to soothe him or herself to sleep. Arousals and brief night wakings are a normative part of the ultradian rhythm of sleep[10] and are not inherently pathologic. However, children who have failed to develop self-soothing skills are often unable to return to sleep independently after these naturally occurring wakings and require parental assistance to return to sleep. If parent intervention is not offered, prolonged night wakings with crying and protest behavior ensue. Behavioral treatment strategies are based on principles of learning and behavior and recruit the parent to act as the agent of change to decrease bedtime problems and frequent night wakings. These strategies include traditional extinction, variations of graduated extinction, and parental education regarding fostering healthy sleep habits.

Traditional or unmodified extinction[11] involves the parent putting the child to bed at bedtime and ignoring the child until a set wake time in the morning while monitoring for safety and/or illness.[12–14] The parent also ignores disruptive behavior that may be displayed by the child, including crying, tantrums, and calling out for the parent. An audio and/or video monitor can be used to ensure the safety of the child while implementing these procedures. It is thought that after the child protests, the combination of sleep pressure and the consistent absence of parental reinforcement will result, over time, in the development of self-soothing skills and the subsequent ability to return to sleep independently. This technique is often referred to as *cry it out* in the public domain.

Although extinction procedures have been demonstrated to be highly effective in teaching children to initiate and maintain sleep without parental assistance, there are several limitations that have been noted in the literature.[14,15] Perhaps most important for parents is that disruptive behaviors (eg, crying, tantrums, calling for parent) typically increase in frequency and severity before improvement (*extinction burst*).[16] Parents must also implement this strategy with consistency and continue to ignore problematic behavior no matter how long the behavior lasts.[14] However, because this procedure can be stressful for parents, many caregivers are unable to use this method with the consistency that is needed to be effective. When implemented inconsistently, parents may actually inadvertently reinforce the disruptive behavior. For example, if parents initially ignore but then eventually respond to the child, thus allowing the child to escape the situation after a certain amount of crying, the child will learn to cry longer the next time to elicit the same response (intermittent reinforcement). Thus, reinforcing the inappropriate behavior may result in protest behaviors that are more severe and intense than before the initial implementation of the extinction procedures. Given the difficulties in implementing standard extinction procedures, there is often a high attrition rate and parental resistance to implementing such a strategy.[17]

Graduated extinction theoretically involves the same underlying process as extinction but involves a more gradual approach. This method is often referred to as *sleep training* or the *checking method*,[18] and parents are instructed to ignore undesired behaviors after bedtime for a specified duration of time while checking in at specific intervals.[11,19] Unlike traditional extinction, some graduated extinction procedures are only implemented at bedtime, and parents are permitted to continue to respond as they typically would if the child wakes during the night. The expectation is that the development of self-soothing skills at bedtime will generalize, making nighttime intervention unnecessary.[20] This strategy has a plethora of empiric support and has also been shown to have better parental adherence and less parental stress when compared with standard extinction.[3,21]

This type of intervention also allows the length of intervals and content of the check-in to be customized to the needs of the family (eg, how long they can tolerate the child's protesting) as well as the child's age, temperament, and developmental level. Check-ins involve the parents comforting the child for a brief amount of time, with a typical range of 15 to 60 seconds. Parents are also encouraged to minimize interaction with their child during this time and may be instructed to repeat the same phrase if they must speak to their child (eg, I love you; it is time to go to sleep).

This practice permits the parent to verbally reassure their child while minimizing attention, as the phrase remains consistent across each interaction. A fixed-interval schedule (eg, every 5 minutes) or a variable-interval schedule (eg, 5 minutes, then 10 minutes, then 15 minutes) can be used in which the interval progressively increases within the same night or across multiple nights. To date, there are no studies that have compared the efficacy of different checking schedules.

Finally, psychoeducational programs that may help to prevent sleep problems from developing provide instruction to expectant parents, as well as parents of infants less than 6 months old, regarding the development of bedtime routines, consistent sleep schedules, parental involvement during sleep initiation, and parental response after spontaneous awakenings during the night. Perhaps most importantly, most programs stress that babies should be put to bed *drowsy but awake* to help them develop the ability to self-soothe at bedtime, thereby enabling them to return to sleep independently after naturally waking during the night. To date, published reviews have concluded that preventative parental sleep education is efficacious and reduces sleep problems,[3,16] with specific studies noting improvements in sleep outcomes.[22–25] However, 2 recent studies found limited efficacy. One study found no impact of an education program provided by nurses in maternity units.[26] This study included an in-hospital education session, phone contacts, and an informational booklet. Note that an earlier pilot study by the same group did find that preventative education was efficacious.[27] Another randomized control trial of a parental intervention with follow-up at 6 months of 554 infants noted efficacy only for improvements in daytime sleep for frequent feeders.[28] This study included parental education provided in a booklet and a DVD with information on such topics as normal infant sleep cycles, crying patterns, and strategies to promote independent settling. No differences were found between the intervention group and a control comparison.

Summary

The behavioral treatments with the most empiric support are unmodified extinction, graduated extinction, and, at least in older studies, preventive parent education,[3,29] with no clear empiric support favoring one approach over another. These 3 strategies are likely most successful because each involves the goal of fostering the development of self-soothing skills in the child. Given the difficulties in implementation and parental acceptance, extinction is likely less often chosen by parents or recommended in clinical practice. In contrast, graduated extinction and preventive education offer a wide range of options that permit a parent and/or treatment provider to customize a protocol to fit the specific needs of a family and to increase parental adherence.

WHAT IS THE BEST AGE TO IMPLEMENT BEHAVIORAL INTERVENTIONS?

Because the sleep of infants changes so rapidly in the first year, practitioners and parents often wonder what the optimal age is for implementation of a behavioral sleep intervention. Furthermore, is there an age when intervention is not recommended (ie, is it ever too late)? Unfortunately, no studies have compared the efficacy or negative effects of behavioral interventions instituted at different ages, such as 3 months vs 6 months. Parenting books make various recommendations, from starting at 12 weeks[30] to letting the child determine when they want to sleep on his or her own.[31] Although there are no data supporting a best age for behavioral interventions for sleep, clinical experience suggests that between 3 to 4 months of age may be a perfect age to implement many aspects of behavioral interventions. For example, this is a good time to transition an infant from a bassinet to a crib, to institute a bedtime routine, and to begin the process of teaching an infant to fall asleep independently. There are certain aspects of sleep physiology that may relate to the timing of behavioral interventions. First of all, 3- to 4-month-old babies are essentially immobile. Although some can roll over, babies at this age are not yet sitting, crawling, pulling to standing, or walking. Thus, the potential disruptive impact of rapid acquisition of motor milestones on sleep is avoided.[32] Additionally, an infant becomes capable of sleep consolidation (ie, the ability to sleep longer stretches of time during the night) by 2 to 3 months of age. One longitudinal study of 75 infants found that sleeping for 8 consecutive hours was most likely to occur at 2 months and sleeping from 10:00 PM to 6:00 AM occurred at 3 months of age.[33] A review of the literature by this same group of investigators found that the greatest rate of change for the longest consolidated sleep period occurs in the first 3 months, with minimal change between 3 and 12 months.[34] They concluded that infants' physiologic ability to sustain sleep develops rapidly in the first few months and that further changes after this time point are related to self-regulation skills, that is, the ability to self-soothe.

In contrast, Douglas and Hill's[35] recent review of behavioral interventions for sleep problems in the first 6 months of life concluded that "the belief that behavioral intervention for sleep in the first 6 months of life improves outcomes for mothers and babies is historically constructed, overlooks feeding problems, and biases interpretation of data."[35] Their review of 43 studies, however, was a mix of a few intervention studies, with the majority being longitudinal studies of infant sleep. Thus, it may not be accurate to conclude that behavioral interventions are ineffective at this young age.

Although Douglas and Hill's[35] review was titled "Behavioral Sleep Interventions in the First Six Months of Life Do Not Improve Outcomes for Mothers or Infants: A Systematic Review," there actually do not seem to be any published studies of behavioral interventions for infants younger than 6 months with identified sleep problems; the only studies that have been conducted are preventative education programs. These programs are not intervention studies per se in that parents are provided with general information during pregnancy or during the first few early months of the infant's life but are not supported in carrying out such interventions in real time.

It is almost never recommended that behavioral sleep interventions be implemented before 3 months of age. Physiologically, newborns may not be ready to sleep for long stretches, often need multiple nighttime feedings, and may not be capable of soothing themselves. In terms of too late, there never seems to be an age at which behavioral interventions are no longer effective and behaviorally based sleep disturbances are no longer malleable to intervention. Several studies have documented success with behavioral interventions with toddlers and preschool-aged children[36–39] and even with school-aged children.[40,41]

Summary

There does not seem to be any research that clearly supports the best age to implement behavioral strategies for sleep disturbances during infancy, either from a preventative or an intervention standpoint. Before 3 months of age is not recommended. The authors propose that an excellent age to learn self-soothing is between 3 and 4 months, although this needs to be customized on an individual basis; overnight feeding should be determined based on the child's growth.

SHOULD SLEEP AIDS AND/OR TRANSITIONAL OBJECTS BE USED AS AN ADJUNCT TO BEHAVIORAL INTERVENTION?

Sleep aids (most often pacifiers) are objects used to promote sleep initiation and maintenance in infants younger than 6 months. Practitioners and parents may question if these items promote or hinder independent sleep behavior. As children reach the ages of 6 to 9 months, sleep aids can be used as a transitional object to provide a sense of comfort and security in the absence of a parent and assist the child in transitioning between waking and sleeping independently. Common examples of sleep aids or transitional objects include pacifiers, blankets, toys, stuffed animals, thumbs for sucking, and/or a clothing item previously worn by a parent.

Cultures that emphasize a child's ability to self-soothe and sleep independently have the highest utilization rates of sleep aids.[42] These items are most commonly seen in Western cultures, especially industrialized societies and in urban areas. It is estimated that 16% to 72% of children between 3 months and 5 years of age make use of a sleep aid to facilitate sleep,[43] and 44% of children between 6 months and 4 years of age use an aid or object specifically at bedtime.[44] Furthermore, the age of the child is also related to the use of a sleep aid, with use increasing from 1 month of age, peaking between 4 and 6 months of age when infants are most likely to sleep independently and be physically able to make use of a sleep aid, and decreasing by 12 months of age.[45,46] For example, one study found that the use of a sleep aid was used by 43% of children at 1 month of age and subsequently declined, with only 26% of infants at 12 months of age using a sleep aid.[45] In addition, of children who used a sleep aid at bedtime, the use of the same object after waking during the night tends to increase with age. That is, infants at 1 month of age used an identical sleep aid for fewer than 30% of awakenings during the night, whereas infants at 6 months, 9 months, and 12 months of age used an identical sleep aid during 60%, 40%, and 50% of wakings, respectively. Finally, the types of sleep aids that are used also changes with age. Infants at 1 month of age are more likely to use a pacifier than at any other age, and infants at 12 months of age tend to use a mix of objects or nothing at all.

It is possible that sleep aids can promote self-soothing skills.[47] Although these are older publications, several studies suggest that children exhibiting self-soothing skills are more likely to use a sleep aid and/or transitional object than children who rely on a parent to transition from wakefulness to sleep.[44,47] Further, infants who use a sleep aid at bedtime and after waking during the night are less likely to exhibit night wakings at 9 months of age.[48] However, an intervention study conducted by Burnham and colleagues[45] found that providing their mother's shirt to 6-month-old infants did not significantly aid in self-soothing at bedtime. It is possible that the tactile characteristics of this transitional object, which may be an important component in identifying an aid or object to promote sleep, were not acceptable. In older children, transitional objects can be quite positive and comforting. For example, a recent study found that a stuffed animal, the huggy puppy, was efficacious in reducing nighttime fears in a study of 104 preschool-aged children (aged 4–6 years).[49]

Clinically, there are potential drawbacks to promoting pacifier use, particularly in children younger than 6 to 7 months. Parents will likely have to replace the pacifier during normative night wakings until the child has the motor skills to retrieve and replace the pacifier during the night. This practice may be similarly problematic with other transitional objects. However, once past this point, sleep aids seem to be beneficial. Thus, parents need to decide what the benefits versus costs of promoting sleep aid use. Finally, the child may replace the pacifier with fingers or a thumb or have significant sleep disruption if the parent stops the pacifier use.

Summary

The use of sleep aids in young children is more common in those able to initiate and maintain sleep independently; however, there is no empiric support for the use of these items either causing or being associated with a change in behavior. Although sleep aids may be successfully used in conjunction with an empirically supported behavioral intervention, the independent presence of a sleep aid is not likely to foster the development of self-soothing skills.

Finally, it is imperative to stress the current recommendations from the American Academy of Pediatrics[50] regarding the sleep environment of a young child. It is advised that a child is put to sleep on his or her back on a firm mattress with a fitted sheet. Soft toys, pillows, blankets, and other stuffed objects or toys should be kept out of the crib. Parents are encouraged to select potential sleep aids with these recommendations in mind.

WHAT IS THE ROLE OF PHARMACOLOGIC AGENTS IN CONJUNCTION WITH BEHAVIORAL INTERVENTION?

Although there are several effective and empirically based behavioral strategies used to treat sleep problems in young children as discussed earlier, pharmacologic interventions may also be used in conjunction with behavioral treatments, as sought out by parents or recommended by physicians. For example, a national survey of 670 community-based pediatricians indicated that the majority had recommended nonprescription medication or prescribed a sleep medication to a child with a sleep problem within the previous 6 months.[51] Approximately 75% of respondents had recommended a nonprescription medication, with antihistamines, such as diphenhydramine, being the most common recommendation; approximately 50% of practitioners had recommended an antihistamine as a sleep intervention for children aged 0 to 2 years. Half of the responding pediatricians had prescribed a sleep medication, with α-receptor agonists the most common prescription, although this was rare in very young children (2%) but more common in 3 to 5 year olds (10%). Overall, 40% of physicians recommended medication for typically developing children with difficulty falling asleep or staying asleep. Although pharmacologic agents are commonly used in clinical practice, it is important for parents and health providers to be aware of the evidence that supports or refutes the use of sedating/hypnotic medications as safe and effective in children.

There are few empiric studies to support the use of prescription or nonprescription medication in the pediatric population.[52,53] In addition, the Food and Drug Administration does not currently approve any medication for the treatment of sleep problems in children. As a result, there is a significant lack of knowledge regarding the effectiveness and safety of the use of these drugs in children. In addition to the obvious concerns regarding safety, there is limited empiric support for pharmacologic agents in the pediatric population, primarily because of a lack of studies. One clinical trial randomly assigned 44 young children aged 6 to 15 months to receive either a placebo or diphenhydramine approximately 30 minutes before bedtime.[54] The results indicated that the groups did not differ in ability to fall asleep independently, sleep latency, number of awakenings during the night, parental happiness or satisfaction, and parental belief that the medication was effective. Essentially, diphenhydramine did not play a role in treating the children's sleep problems; the trial was discontinued before completion. In contrast, an older study[12] evaluated the effects of combining extinction and sedative medication (trimeprazine tartrate), prescribed in a reducing dose over the first 10 days of extinction in a sample of 45 children, aged 7 to 27 months. The combined extinction/medication group was found to have abrupt improvements in sleep, whereas the extinction and placebo groups had slow improvements. Finally, a recent meta-analysis of the use of melatonin in the treatment of sleep disturbances in children with autism spectrum disorders found overall efficacy; but none of these studies were conducted with children younger than 3 years, and most did not do so in combination with a behavioral intervention.[55]

Summary

Behavioral treatment approaches for young children with difficulty falling asleep and/or staying asleep are well supported in the literature and should be the primary treatment modality in this population. The American Academy of Sleep Medicine's multidisciplinary task force on Pharmacotherapy in Pediatric Sleep Medicine stresses the importance and effectiveness of behavioral strategies as the primary intervention.[52] If pharmacologic agents are used at all, they should be as an adjunct to and in combination with empirically supported behavioral treatment. Only in specific situations, such as if the safety or welfare of the child is threatened, there is an acute stressor, or the family is too stressed to manage the implementation of behavioral changes, should medications be used to treat sleep problems in typically developing children. Additional studies are clearly needed to assess the role of pharmacologic treatments as an adjunct to behavioral interventions.

ARE BEHAVIORAL INTERVENTIONS MORE HELPFUL OR HARMFUL?

Although no systematic negative effects of sleep training have been supported by research, the potential iatrogenic effect of behavioral approaches to childhood sleep problems continues to be a controversial area. Although there is a solid empiric foundation demonstrating that behavioral approaches improve children's sleep,[3] there continues to be discussion as to whether such approaches cause harm in other domains of child and family functioning. Reviews and opinion pieces representing both sides of the issue continue to be published and receive significant attention.[56,57]

Overall, there are few studies investigating secondary outcomes of behavioral approaches; no studies to date have started with a priori hypotheses that negative effects would occur. In the most comprehensive longitudinal study to date,[58,59] a follow-up study at 6 years of age was conducted following a randomized controlled trial of an individual behavioral sleep intervention delivered by nurses to infants (8–10 months) with an identified sleep problem and their mothers. Of the 326 initial participants, 225 participated in the follow-up at 6 years of age (63%). The overall findings were that behavioral interventions for infant sleep improve sleep in the short-term with no long-term negative effects. More specifically, there were no negative effects on child mental health, psychosocial functioning, the parent-child relationship, maternal mental health, or parenting style in children receiving the behavioral intervention compared with the control group.

A recent article by Moore and Mindell[60] provides a comprehensive review of pediatric behavioral sleep intervention studies with inclusion of secondary outcomes (N = 35) and looked at the effects on the child, on the parent, and on the parent-child relationship. The conclusion of this review was that there were no systematic negative effects of any behavioral sleep interventions. If anything, only positive effects of these interventions were found. A brief review of the main outcomes is provided here.

Effects on the Child

Studies including child-based secondary outcomes have included measures of mood, temperament, and daytime behavior/functioning. In terms of research on child mood following behavioral sleep interventions, research is scarce. One study with a pre-post design investigated infant mood in 33 infants who were part of an inpatient behavioral sleep intervention at 6 to 23 months of age.[61] At 2 months after the intervention, 15 of 19 infants who were initially described as "irritable" before the intervention were described as happier, more playful, calmer, more cheerful, and easy to please. The two studies that have assessed the impact of sleep interventions on child temperament, not surprisingly, did not find any impact.[61–63]

Most of the research on secondary outcomes of behavioral sleep intervention has targeted daytime behavior/functioning of the child. Although most studies have not included children with clinically significant behavior problems, several did describe positive changes in behavior. For example, Seymour and colleagues[64] found that sleep improvements related to positive changes in daytime behavior, including being happier, easier to handle, and less aggressive. France[65] found improvements in agreeableness, likeability, and emotionality up to 18 months after the intervention in 35 infants (6–24 months) compared with controls. Other studies have also found improvements in daytime behaviors, including both internalizing and externalizing behaviors.[63,66]

Parent Effects

Although not the focus of this article, child sleep affects parent sleep; improvements in child sleep have been found to relate to improvements in parent sleep quality and lower fatigue levels[38,67,68] as well as decreased night wakings.[20] Studies have also found improvements in parent well-being (eg, stress, distress, mood, marital satisfaction) with improvements in the child's sleep.[63,68]

Parent-Child Relationship

Both in the popular press[69] and in academic journals,[56] concerns have been raised about the impact of behavioral sleep training on the parent-child relationship. Studies have not only failed to support any negative outcomes but have also identified potential benefits. For example, following a behavioral sleep intervention with 8 to 10 month olds, one study found 84% of mothers reported that behavioral interventions had a positive affect on their relationship with their child.[70] Two studies have specifically looked at infant security as a primary outcome of a behavioral sleep intervention and found a significant improvement in security at day 3 of the intervention and further improvements notes at week 6 of treatment.[12,65] No improvements in security were found in controls or untreated infants. A third study compared 95 infants referred for a sleep problem with a community comparison and found significant improvements in security after the intervention.[37] Group differences in security (with infants with a sleep problem described as less secure) found at baseline were eliminated following the intervention.

Summary

Although behavioral sleep interventions may be difficult for parents to implement and, in some cases, may involve the child protesting in the short-term, no studies to date have found any negative effects on the child. Based on existing research, clinicians can confidently recommend behavioral interventions without fear of short- or long-term harmful effects in the child or family.

SUMMARY

Sleep problems in young children are prevalent and may become chronic without treatment. Behavioral interventions are clearly effective; but questions still remain and controversies exist, which provide barriers to implementing these interventions. Overall, the results of empiric studies as well as clinical experience suggest there is no perfect or one-size-fits-all intervention but rather that these strategies need to be tailored to the individual child and family. Research does not support the best age to implement behavioral strategies, although the authors postulate that 3 to 4 months of age may be optimal in many cases. Parents should aim to improve sleep behavior as soon as a problem has been identified and when they feel comfortable using intervention procedures to modify the behavior of the child. The practice of pairing sleep aids with an evidence-based behavioral treatment strategy also has some empiric support. However, there are few data supporting the use of sedative/hypnotic pharmacologic agents in children either alone or in combination with behavioral treatments; these agents should be used, if at all, with caution and only under the supervision of a health care provider. Finally, parents can be assured that research does not indicate a link between behavioral approaches used to improve the sleep in young children and any negative effects on the child, parent, or child-parent relationship outcomes.

REFERENCES

1. Liu X, Liu L, Owens JA, et al. Sleep patterns and sleep problems among schoolchildren in the United States and China. Pediatrics 2005;115: 241–9.
2. Mindell JA, Owens JA. A clinical guide to pediatric sleep: diagnosis and management of sleep problems. 2nd edition. Philadelphia: Lippincott Williams & Wilkins; 2009.
3. Mindell JA, Kuhn B, Lewin DS, et al, American Academy of Sleep Medicine. Behavioral treatment of bedtime problems and night wakings in infants and young children. Sleep 2006;29:1263–76.
4. Sadeh A, Mindell JA, Luedtke K, et al. Sleep and sleep ecology in the first 3 years: a web-based study. J Sleep Res 2009;18:60–73.
5. Byars KC, Yolton K, Rausch J, et al. Prevalence, patterns, and persistence of sleep problems in the first 3 years of life. Pediatrics 2012;129: e276–84.
6. Beebe DW. Cognitive, behavioral, and functional consequences of inadequate sleep in children and adolescents. Pediatr Clin North Am 2011;58: 649–65.
7. Fallone G, Acebo C, Seifer R, et al. Experimental restriction of sleep opportunity in children: effects on teacher ratings. Sleep 2005;28:1279–85.
8. Hart CN, Cairns A, Jelalian E. Sleep and obesity in children and adolescents. Pediatr Clin North Am 2011;58:715–33.
9. Mindell JA, Owens J, Alves R, et al. Give children and adolescents the gift of a good night's sleep: a call to action. Sleep Med 2011;12:203–4.
10. Sadeh A. Assessment of intervention for infant night waking: parental reports and activity-based home monitoring. J Consult Clin Psychol 1994;62: 63–8.
11. Ferber R. Solve your child's sleep problems. New York: Simon & Schuster; 1985.
12. France KG, Blampied NM, Wilkinson P. Treatment of infant sleep disturbance by trimeprazine in

combination with extinction. J Dev Behav Pediatr 1991;12:308–14.

13. Rickert VI, Johnson CM. Reducing nocturnal awakening and crying episodes in infants and young children: a comparison between scheduled awakenings and systematic ignoring. Pediatrics 1988; 81:203–12.

14. Reid M, Walter AL, O'Leary SG. Treatment of young children's bedtime refusal and nighttime wakings: a comparison of "standard" and graduated ignoring procedures. J Abnorm Child Psychol 1999;27:5–16.

15. France KG, Hudson SM. Behavior management of infant sleep disturbance. J Appl Behav Anal 1990; 23:91–8.

16. Kuhn BR, Elliott AJ. Treatment efficacy in behavioral pediatric sleep medicine. J Psychosom Res 2003;54:587–97.

17. Borkowski MM, Hunter KE, Johnson CM. White noise and scheduled bedtime routines to reduce infant and childhood sleep disturbances. Behav Ther (N Y N Y) 2001;24:29–37.

18. Mindell JA. Sleeping through the night: how infants, toddlers, and their parents can get a good night's sleep. New York: Harper Collins; 2005.

19. Richman N, Douglas J, Hunt H. Behavioural methods in the treatment of sleep disorders - a pilot study. J Child Psychol Psychiatry 1985;26:581–90.

20. Mindell JA, Durand VM. Treatment of childhood sleep disorders: generalization across disorders and effects on family members. J Pediatr Psychol 1993;18:731–50.

21. Hiscock H, Wake M. Randomised controlled trial of behavioural infant sleep intervention to improve infant sleep and maternal mood. BMJ 2002;324: 1062–5.

22. Adachi Y, Sato C, Nishino N, et al. A brief parental education for shaping sleep habits in 4-month-old infants. Clin Med Res 2009;7:85–92.

23. Adair R, Zuckerman B, Bauchner H, et al. Reducing night waking in infancy: a primary care intervention. Pediatrics 1992;89:585–8.

24. Wolfson A, Lacks P, Futterman A. Effects of parent training on infant sleeping patterns, parents' stress, and perceived parental competence. J Consult Clin Psychol 1992;60:41–8.

25. St James-Roberts I, Sleep J, Morris S, et al. Use of a behavioural programme in the first 3 months to prevent infant crying and sleeping problems. J Paediatr Child Health 2001;37:289–97.

26. Stremler R, Hodnett E, Kenton L, et al. Effect of behavioural-educational intervention on sleep for primiparous women and their infants in early postpartum: multisite randomised controlled trial. BMJ 2013;346:f1164.

27. Stremler R, Hodnett E, Lee K, et al. A behavioral-education intervention to promote maternal and infant sleep: a pilot randomized controlled trial. Sleep 2006;29:1609–15.

28. Hiscock H, Cook F, Bayer J, et al. Preventing early infant sleep and crying problems and postnatal depression: a randomized trial. Pediatrics 2014; 133(2):e346–54.

29. Kuhn BR, Weidinger D. Interventions for infant and toddler sleep disturbance: a review. Child Fam Behav Ther 2000;22:33–50.

30. Giordano S. Twelve hours' sleep by twelve weeks old: a step-by-step plan for baby sleep success. New York: Dutton; 2006.

31. Sears W, Sears M. The attachment parenting book: a commonsense guide to understanding and nurturing your baby. New York: Little, Brown and Company; 2001.

32. Scher A. The onset of upright locomotion and night wakings. Percept Mot Skills 1996;83:1122.

33. Henderson JM, France KG, Owens JL, et al. Sleeping through the night: the consolidation of self-regulated sleep across the first year of life. Pediatrics 2010;126:e1081–7.

34. Henderson JM, France KG, Blampied NM. The consolidation of infants' nocturnal sleep across the first year of life. Sleep Med Rev 2011;15: 211–20.

35. Douglas PS, Hill PS. Behavioral sleep interventions in the first six months of life do not improve outcomes for mothers or infants: a systematic review. J Dev Behav Pediatr 2013;34:497–507.

36. Blunden S. Behavioural treatments to encourage solo sleeping in pre-school children: an alternative to controlled crying. J Child Health Care 2011;15: 107–17.

37. Eckerberg B. Treatment of sleep problems in families with young children: effects of treatment on family well-being. Acta Paediatr 2004;93: 126–34.

38. Mindell JA, Telofski LS, Wiegand B, et al. A nightly bedtime routine: impact on sleep problems in young children and maternal mood. Sleep 2009; 32:599–606.

39. Moore BA, Friman PC, Fruzzetti AE, et al. Brief report: evaluating the Bedtime Pass Program for child resistance to bedtime–a randomized, controlled trial. J Pediatr Psychol 2007;32:283–7.

40. Adkins KW, Molloy C, Weiss SK, et al. Effects of a standardized pamphlet on insomnia in children with autism spectrum disorders. Pediatrics 2012; 130(Suppl 2):S139–44.

41. Paine S, Gradisar G. A randomised controlled trial of cognitive-behaviour therapy for behavioural insomnia of childhood in school-aged children. Behav Res Ther 2011;49:379–88.

42. Jenni OG, O'Connor BB. Children's sleep: an interplay between culture and biology. Pediatrics 2005; 115:204–16.

43. Passman RH, Halonen JS. A developmental survey of young children's attachments to inanimate objects. J Genet Psychol 1979;134:165–78.

44. Wolf AW, Lozoff B. Object attachment, thumb-sucking, and the passage to sleep. J Am Acad Child Adolesc Psychiatry 1989;28:287–92.

45. Burnham MM, Goodlin-Jones BL, Gaylor EE, et al. Nighttime sleep-wake patterns and self-soothing from birth to one year of age: a longitudinal intervention study. J Child Psychol Psychiatry 2002; 43:713–25.

46. Burnham MM, Goodlin-Jones BL, Gaylor EE, et al. Use of sleep aids during the first year of life. Pediatrics 2002;109:594–601.

47. Anders TF, Halpern LF, Hua J. Sleeping through the night: a developmental perspective. Pediatrics 1992;90:554–60.

48. Paret I. Night waking and its relationship to mother-infant interaction in nine-month-old infants. In: Call J, Galenson E, Tyson R, editors. Frontiers of infant psychiatry. New York: Basic Books; 1983. p. 171–7.

49. Kushnir J, Sadeh A. Assessment of brief interventions for nighttime fears in preschool children. Eur J Pediatr 2012;171:67–75.

50. Section on Pediatric Pulmonology, Subcommittee on Obstructive Sleep Apnea Syndrome. American Academy of Pediatrics. Clinical practice guideline: diagnosis and management of childhood obstructive sleep apnea syndrome. Pediatrics 2002;109: 704–12.

51. Owens JA, Rosen CL, Mindell JA. Medication use in the treatment of pediatric insomnia: results of a survey of community-based pediatricians. Pediatrics 2003;111:e628–35.

52. Owens JA, Babcock D, Blumer J, et al. The use of pharmacotherapy in the treatment of pediatric insomnia in primary care: rational approaches. A consensus meeting summary. J Clin Sleep Med 2005;1:49–59.

53. Mindell JA, Emslie G, Blumer J, et al. Pharmacologic management of insomnia in children and adolescents: consensus statement. Pediatrics 2006; 117:e1223–32.

54. Merenstein D, Diener-West M, Halbower AC, et al. The trial of infant response to diphenhydramine: the TIRED study–a randomized, controlled, patient-oriented trial. Arch Pediatr Adolesc Med 2006;160:707–12.

55. Rossignol DA, Frye RE. Melatonin in autism spectrum disorders: a systematic review and meta-analysis. Dev Med Child Neurol 2011;53: 783–92.

56. Blunden SL, Thompson KR, Dawson D. Behavioural sleep treatments and night time crying in infants: challenging the status quo. Sleep Med Rev 2011;15:327–34.

57. Sadeh A, Mindell JA, Owens J. Why care about sleep of infants and their parents? Sleep Med Rev 2011;15:335–7.

58. Price A, Wake M, Ukoumunne OC, et al. Outcomes at six years of age for children with infant sleep problems: longitudinal community-based study. Sleep Med 2012;13(8):991–8.

59. Price A, Wake M, Ukoumunne OC, et al. Five-year follow-up of harms and benefits of behavioral infant sleep intervention: randomized trial. Pediatrics 2012;130:643–51.

60. Moore M, Mindell JA. The impact of behavioral interventions for sleep problems on secondary outcomes in young children and their families. In: Wolfson A, Montgomery-Downs H, editors. The Oxford handbook of infant, child, and adolescent sleep and behavior. New York: Oxford University Press; 2013. p. 547–58.

61. Skuladottir A, Thome M. Changes in infant sleep problems after a family-centered intervention. Pediatr Nurs 2003;29:375–8.

62. Pinilla T, Birch LL. Help me make it through the night: behavioral entrainment of breast-fed infants' sleep patterns. Pediatrics 1993;91:436–44.

63. Hiscock H, Bayer J, Gold L, et al. Improving infant sleep and maternal mental health: a cluster randomised trial. Arch Dis Child 2007;92:952–8.

64. Seymour FW, Bayfield G, Brock P, et al. Management of night-waking in young children. Aust J Fam Ther 1983;4:217–23.

65. France KG. Behavior characteristics and security in sleep-disturbed infants treated with extinction. J Pediatr Psychol 1992;17:467–75.

66. Minde K, Faucon A, Falkner S. Sleep problems in toddlers: effects of treatment on their daytime behavior. J Am Acad Child Adolesc Psychiatry 1994;33:1114–21.

67. Hall WA, Clauson M, Carty EM, et al. Effects on parents of an intervention to resolve infant behavioral sleep problems. Pediatr Nurs 2006;32:243–50.

68. Mindell JA, Du Mond C, Sadeh A, et al. Efficacy of an Internet-based intervention for infant and toddler sleep disturbances. Sleep 2011;34:451–8.

69. Narvaez D. Dangers of "crying it out": damaging children and their relationships for the long-term. Psychol Today. Available at: http://www.psychologytoday.com/blog/moral-landscapes/201112/dangers-crying-it-out2011.

70. Hiscock H, Bayer JK, Hampton A, et al. Long-term mother and child mental health effects of a population-based infant sleep intervention: cluster-randomized, controlled trial. Pediatrics 2008;122: e621–7.

Cognitive-Behavioral Therapy for Comorbid Insomnia and Chronic Pain

Patrick H. Finan, PhD*, Luis F. Buenaver, PhD,
Virginia T. Runko, PhD, Michael T. Smith, PhD

KEYWORDS

• Insomnia • Chronic pain • Comorbid • Cognitive-behavioral therapy for insomnia

KEY POINTS

• Cognitive-behavioral therapy for insomnia (CBT-I) for comorbid insomnia and chronic pain demonstrates clinically meaningful improvements in sleep symptoms, particularly sleep continuity.
• CBT-I for comorbid insomnia and chronic pain does not consistently improve pain severity, but appears to reduce pain interference and disability in several studies.
• Hybrid interventions that target both pain and insomnia have demonstrated feasibility in small pilot samples, but further conclusions must be deferred until a larger trial is reported.
• More comprehensive and dynamic pain assessment strategies may reveal effects for CBT-I and hybrid interventions not captured through single-occasion pain severity measures.

INTRODUCTION

Most patients with chronic pain report poor sleep quality. Insomnia, the most prevalent form of sleep disturbance in chronic pain, may directly contribute to poor long-term outcomes by affecting multiple dimensions of chronic pain pathophysiology and psychosocial functioning. Sleep loss impairs immune function,[1,2] emotion regulation,[3,4] and cognitive function,[5,6] and heightens pain sensitivity.[7] These processes are considered both vulnerabilities to and consequences of chronic pain.[8–11] As such, there is a growing interest in the development and evaluation of sleep-related interventions among patients with chronic pain and in individuals at risk for developing chronic pain.

Treating sleep disturbance in patients with chronic pain is of interest for several reasons. First, a recent systematic review indicates that psychological and pharmacologic strategies for chronic pain management show only modest effects in reducing pain and pain-related disability.[12]

Targeting additional symptom clusters that may actively contribute to chronic pain severity and persistence, such as sleep disturbance, may be necessary to improve pain-management outcomes. Furthermore, and perhaps somewhat surprisingly, recent prospective studies using rigorous statistical methodologies have suggested that in some idiopathic pain conditions, such as temporomandibular joint disorder,[13] sleep disturbance might in fact be a more robust predictor of subsequent pain than vice versa. A recent laboratory study demonstrated that extension of sleep among individuals with mild chronic sleep loss was associated with reduced pain sensitivity.[14] Thus, it is reasonable to hypothesize that interventions that target sleep in patients with chronic pain may produce improvements in pain symptoms as insomnia dissipates.

Cognitive-behavioral therapy for insomnia (CBT-I) is the standard of care for treating chronic primary insomnia. The efficacy of CBT-I in primary insomnia is comparable with that of modern sedative

Department of Psychiatry and Behavioral Sciences, Johns Hopkins University School of Medicine, Baltimore, MD, USA
* Corresponding author.
E-mail address: pfinan1@jhu.edu

Sleep Med Clin 9 (2014) 261–274
http://dx.doi.org/10.1016/j.jsmc.2014.02.007
1556-407X/14/$ – see front matter © 2014 Elsevier Inc. All rights reserved.

hypnotics, with the advantages of long-term sustainability of treatment effects[15,16] and a favorable side-effect profile.[17] CBT-I is standardized, and can be implemented in a wide range of outpatient settings and formats.[18–21] In the past decade, CBT-I has increasingly been investigated for the treatment of insomnia occurring in the context of medical and psychiatric comorbidities, with promising results.[22] Most of these studies limited their primary outcomes to sleep parameters. A handful of researchers, however, have recently begun to study the effects of CBT-I on sleep and pain-related outcomes. The theoretical frameworks and some of the coping skills taught in CBT-I overlap with the skills taught in cognitive-behavioral therapy for pain (CBT-P), but the 2 treatments also retain many distinct pain-related and sleep-related components. There is a potential for skills taught in CBT-I to improve pain-related outcomes despite a primary focus on insomnia. In addition, it is reasonable to hypothesize that the components of CBT-I and CBT-P may be blended into a hybrid intervention format that works synergistically on sleep and pain symptoms. Both of these possibilities have been tested in preliminary randomized controlled trials (RCTs), which are the focus of this article. The objectives of this review are to: (1) summarize the findings of this first wave of published clinical trials; (2) discuss the limitations; and (3) identify promising directions for the next wave of studies.

CBT-I FOR COMORBID INSOMNIA AND CHRONIC PAIN

CBT-I is most commonly practiced as a multicomponent treatment that uses a variety of behavioral interventions and cognitive restructuring approaches. It is a short-term intervention that is typically conducted over 4 to 8 individual or group sessions. The most commonly used therapeutic elements include: (1) general sleep education; (2) the application of operant and classical conditioning principles via stimulus control instructions; (3) the replacement of sleep-interfering behaviors with sleep-promoting behaviors through sleep-hygiene education and behavior-change counseling; (4) relaxation training (eg, deep breathing, guided imagery); (5) the alteration of circadian regularity and alignment; (6) the manipulation of homeostatic sleep drive to consolidate sleep via sleep restriction[23]; and (7) the use of cognitive therapy techniques to modify maladaptive sleep-related cognitions. Much of the therapy is data driven, relying on the patient's self-monitoring of daily sleeping patterns, including time in bed (TIB), sleep onset latency (SOL), wake after sleep onset (WASO), and total sleep time (TST).

Currie and Colleagues

Primary findings

The first RCT of CBT-I for patients with comorbid insomnia and chronic pain (N = 60) compared seven 2-hour CBT-I group sessions held weekly with a self-monitoring/wait-list control.[24] The components of therapy followed traditional CBT-I guidelines (**Table 1**), with one notable modification: the contribution of pain to sleep problems was specifically addressed through guided readings and group discussion. The investigators found that patients in the CBT-I condition demonstrated significant improvements in daily diary–measured SOL, sleep efficiency (SE), WASO, and sleep quality. These effects were maintained at the 3-month follow-up assessment. Actigraphic measures of nocturnal physical activity were also significantly reduced in the CBT-I condition. Of note, however, pain severity ratings did not significantly improve.

Analysis

This study[24] established that CBT-I may produce clinically significant changes in self-reported and actigraphy-measured sleep for patients with insomnia and comorbid chronic pain. The use of a wait-list control condition, however, significantly tempers the strength of this conclusion, because of the strong expectation for minimal improvement created by randomization to a wait list. That pain was not significantly reduced in the CBT-I group raises the possibility that clinical improvements in sleep do not directly lead to reductions in pain severity. However, methodological constraints may limit this interpretation. First, participants were selected on the basis of having insomnia symptoms that developed secondary to chronic pain, and information about their pain status before the development of insomnia was not available. Because it is not possible to determine if and to what extent the development of insomnia symptoms altered pre-existing pain symptoms in this sample, one cannot conclude that the lack of pain changes following treatment of insomnia necessarily indicate that CBT-I is inefficacious for pain symptoms. Rather, it could be that the pain symptoms, by virtue of having preceded the development of insomnia symptoms, were not being maintained by insomnia and therefore were not influenced by improvements in insomnia symptoms. This possibility could be evaluated in future studies by assessing time-contingent dependencies between insomnia and pain symptoms through daily diaries before and after treatment. A second limitation is that pain severity was the only pain-related outcome measured, and was considered a secondary outcome; a wider range of pain-related outcomes that measure the multidimensional nature of pain (eg, pain interference, pain catastrophizing) would be necessary to adequately evaluate the broader influence of CBT-I on pain-related outcomes. Third, although groups did not significantly differ from pretreatment to posttreatment on changes in pain, the means trended in this direction. The between-groups effect size (Cohen's d[25]) of CBT-I versus Control on pain was 0.51 at posttreatment and 0.64 at the 3-month follow-up. These values are considered medium effect sizes.[25] As a point of comparison, a recent meta-analysis of the effect of CBT-P shows small to medium effect sizes on pain severity, disability, and catastrophizing at posttreatment, with even smaller effects at follow-up.[12,26] That reductions in pain severity were observed (though not to the point of statistical significance) by Currie and colleagues[24] at 3 months for the CBT-I group might be considered clinically relevant, and raises the issue of whether longer-term follow-up periods are needed to realize the full effect of CBT-I on pain and pain-related outcomes.

Rybarczyk and Colleagues

Primary findings
Expanding on the study by Currie and colleagues,[24] Rybarczyk and colleagues[27] compared CBT-I (n = 23) with a stress-management and wellness control (n = 28) in a subsample of patients with comorbid insomnia and osteoarthritis (OA). The CBT-I intervention (see **Table 1**) did not specifically address pain interference with sleep, and the OA patients participated in group sessions along with patients with other nonpainful medical conditions. The focus here is on the data for the OA/pain subsample only. Results indicated that, relative to the stress-management control, CBT-I significantly improved daily diary–reported SE, WASO, and SOL.[28] Pain on the McGill Pain Questionnaire (MPQ[29]), which measures both sensory and affective components of pain, was not significantly reduced by the CBT-I intervention. However, a follow-up analysis[28] revealed that CBT-I patients reported significantly less pain on the SF-36 Bodily Pain scale[30] at posttreatment, and tended to maintain those benefits at 1-year follow-up (P = .08).

Analysis
By including an active control condition, this study[27] permitted a more rigorous test of CBT-I against a stress management control with similar cognitive demand and expectancy characteristics. Overall, the findings from this study confirmed the efficacy of CBT-I for self-reported sleep-related outcomes in patients with comorbid chronic pain and insomnia. Findings on pain-related measures were equivocal, perhaps owing to differences in measurement. The MPQ assesses sensory and affective characteristics of the pain experience, whereas the SF-36 is a measure that includes items measuring both pain severity and interference in function.[30] Similar to the study by Currie and colleagues,[24] this study was primarily focused on sleep-related outcomes, and lacked a comprehensive pain-assessment strategy. Nonetheless, the superiority of CBT-I over an active control on primary sleep outcomes offers compelling support for its efficacy in treating sleep among patients with insomnia and comorbid chronic pain.

Edinger and Colleagues

Primary findings
Similar CBT-I benefits were observed in a small RCT involving patients with comorbid fibromyalgia and insomnia.[31] Clinically significant improvements in daily diary SE and TST were observed in 43% (6 of 14) of CBT-I patients compared with 7% (1 of 15) in a control condition receiving only sleep-hygiene education, and in 0 of 7 in a usual-care condition. Objective actigraphic measures of sleep yielded comparable results, including shorter mean SOL and lower variability across days in both SOL and TST, suggesting that sleep became more reliable following CBT-I, an underappreciated but common outcome associated with CBT-I. Across most sleep outcomes, treatment gains were maintained at 6-month follow-up. Significant differences between the CBT-I and control groups were not observed for pain outcomes (ie, severity and sensory/affective pain), although means trended in that direction and effect sizes between the CBT-I and usual-care groups at postintervention were medium to large (Cohen d 0.51 and 1.74 for pain severity[32] and sensory/affective pain,[29] respectively). Of interest, patients in the sleep-hygiene group scored significantly differently to usual-care controls on both pain severity and sensory/affective pain measures. Subgroup analyses indicated that the association of sleep-hygiene treatment and pain-related improvements was driven by a portion of patients in the sleep-hygiene group who self-initiated the behavioral strategy of standardizing their sleep times and achieved a 25% or greater reduction in TIB variability. This subgroup showed a significantly greater reduction in self-reported sensory/affective pain than usual-care controls.

Analysis
Overall, the results of this study[31] suggest that CBT-I may be an effective intervention for patients with fibromyalgia, as it provided favorable results

Table 1
Comparison of CBT-I and hybrid clinical trials for comorbid insomnia and chronic pain

				Studies in Which CBT-I Was the Active Treatment						
Authors,[Ref.] Year	Treatment Type	Study Sample	PSG Exclusion Criteria	Active Treatment Components	Treatment Duration	Treatment Format	Pain Measures	Sleep Measures	Significant CBT-Related Improvements in Pain?	Significant CBT-Related Improvements in Sleep?
Currie et al,[24] 2000	CBT-I vs wait-list control	Chronic nonmalignant pain + insomnia N = 60	PSG not administered	GSE; SCT; SRT; SHE; RT, CT Pain coping education	7 weekly sessions; 2 h/session	Group; 5–7 patients/group	MPI	Daily diary; actigraphy; PSQI	No	Yes 1. Diary SOL, SE, WASO 2. Sleep quality 3. Nocturnal activity
Rybarczyk et al,[27] 2005; Vitiello et al,[28] 2009	CBT-I vs stress management control	Osteoarthritis + insomnia N = 51	AHI <15 PLMI <30	SCT; SRT; SHE; RT; CT	8 weekly sessions; 2 h/session	Group; 5 patients/group	MPQ; SF-36 Bodily Pain	Daily Diary	Yes 1. SF-36 Bodily Pain	Yes 1. Diary SOL; SE; WASO
Edinger et al,[31] 2005	CBT-I vs sleep-hygiene control vs usual care	Fibromyalgia + insomnia N = 47	AHI <15 PLMI <15	GSE; SCT; SRT	6 weekly sessions; 45–60 min in week 1, 15–30 min in weeks 2–6	Individual	MPQ; BPI	Daily diary; actigraphy; ISQ	No	Yes 1. Diary SOL; SE; TWT 2. Actigraphy SOL and SOL variability; TST variability 3. Insomnia Severity
Jungquist et al,[35] 2010; Jungquist et al,[38] 2012	CBT-I vs contact control	Chronic nonmalignant pain + insomnia N = 28	AHI <10 PLM not specified	SCT; SRT; SHE; CT	8 weekly sessions; 30–60 min/session	Individual	Daily diary; MPQ; MPI; PDI	Daily diary; ISI; ESS	Yes 1. Pain interference (MPI)	Yes 1. Diary SOL; SE; WASO; awakenings 2. Insomnia Severity

Studies in Which a Hybrid CBT-I/-P Was the Active Treatment

Authors,[Ref.] Year	Treatment Types	Study Population	Active Treatment Components	Treatment Duration	Treatment Format	Pain Measures	Sleep Measures	Significant Hybrid Treatment-Related Improvements in Pain?	Significant Hybrid Treatment-Related Improvements in Sleep?
Pigeon et al,[40] 2012	Hybrid CBT-I/-P vs CBT-I vs CBT-P vs wait-list control	Chronic nonmalignant pain + insomnia N = 21 AHI <10 PLMI not specified	GSE; SCT; SRT; SHE; RT; sleep-related CT; sleep-related relapse prevention; pain education; pain-related CT; activity pacing; problem solving; communication skills training; pain-related relapse prevention	10 weekly sessions; session time not reported	Individual	MPI; PDI	Daily diary; ISI; ESS	No	Yes 1. Insomnia Severity[a]
Tang et al,[41] 2012	Hybrid CBT-I/-P vs symptom monitoring control	Chronic nonmalignant pain + insomnia N = 20 PSG not administered	GSE; SCT; SRT; CT; pain education; behavioral activation; pain-related CT	4 weekly sessions; 2 h/session	Individual	Daily diary; BPI; CISP; PSPS	Daily diary; actigraphy; ISI; DBAS; PSAS; APSQ	Yes 1. Pain Interference (BPI)	Yes 1. Insomnia Severity (ISI) 2. Diary SOL; SE; WASO; TST

(continued on next page)

Table 1
(continued)

Studies in Which a Hybrid CBT-I/-P Was the Active Treatment

Authors,[Ref.] Year	Treatment Types	Study Population	Active Treatment Components	Treatment Duration	Treatment Format	Pain Measures	Sleep Measures	Significant Hybrid Treatment-Related Improvements in Pain?	Significant Hybrid Treatment-Related Improvements in Sleep?
Vitiello et al,[42] 2013	Hybrid CBT-I/P vs CBT-P vs Education	Chronic osteoarthritis and insomnia	PSG not administered SHE; SCT; SRT; pain education; behavioral activation; relaxation; activity pacing; imagery; pain-related CT	6 weekly session; 90 min/session	Groups; 5–12/group	Graded Chronic Pain Scale; arthritis symtpoms	ISI; Actigraphy SE	No	Yes 1. ISI 2. SE

Abbreviations: APSQ, Anxiety and Preoccupation about Sleep Questionnaire; BPI, Brief Pain Inventory; CBT, cognitive-behavioral therapy; CBT-I, cognitive-behavioral therapy for insomnia; CBT-P, cognitive-behavioral therapy for pain; CISP, Catastrophizing in Pain Scale; CT, cognitive therapy; DBAS, Dysfunctional Beliefs About Sleep Scale; ESS, Epworth Sleepiness Scale; GSE, general sleep education; ISI, Insomnia Severity Index; ISQ, Insomnia Symptom Questionnaire; MPI, Multidimensional Pain Inventory; MPQ, McGill Pain Questionnaire; PDI, Pain Disability Index; PSAS, Presleep Arousal Scale; PSPS, Pain Self-Perception Scale; PSQI, Pittsburgh Sleep Quality Index; RT, relaxation training; SCT, stimulus control therapy; SE, sleep efficiency; SF-36, 36-item Short-Form Survey; SHE, sleep-hygiene education; SII, Sleep Impairment Index; SOL, sleep onset latency; SRT, sleep restriction therapy; TST, total sleep time; TWT, total wake time; WASO, wake after sleep onset.

a The hybrid group evidenced a larger effect size than CBT-I, but was not significantly different after adjusting for multiple comparisons.

on both subjective and objective sleep criteria. However, as with prior studies in other chronic nonmalignant pain populations, the results were equivocal with respect to the efficacy of CBT-I for reducing pain and pain-related symptoms. Fibromyalgia pain may be substantively different from pain associated with osteoarthritis and other types of degenerative musculoskeletal disorders, so it is difficult to compare general pain measures across studies. Future efforts with this population could expand outcome measures to include fibromyalgia-specific measures, such as a body map or the Fibromyalgia Impact Questionnaire.[33] Furthermore, because nonrestorative sleep is such a prevalent complaint among patients with fibromyalgia,[34] it would be important to know if CBT-I improvements in SOL, SE, and TST are associated with improvements in the perception of restorative sleep.

Jungquist and Colleagues

Primary findings
Another RCT[35] of patients with chronic nonmalignant back and/or neck pain and comorbid insomnia found that, relative to a contact control (n = 9), CBT-I (n = 19) produced significant posttreatment improvements in daily diary–reported SOL, SE, WASO, number of awakenings, insomnia severity, and pain interference measured with the Multidimensional Pain Inventory.[36] CBT-I did not significantly improve posttreatment daily diary–reported pain severity or pain disability measured with the Pain Disability Index.[37] Although TST was not significantly enhanced at posttreatment, which is commonly the case among interventions that include sleep restriction, clinically and statistically significant gains in TST (23 minutes) were observed at 6-month follow-up.[38] In addition, posttreatment reductions in pain interference were maintained at both 3-month and 6-month follow-up periods, providing preliminary evidence for the sustainability of CBT-I effects on a key functional pain-related outcome.

Analysis
The multimodal (ie, diary and single-occasion measurement), multidimensional (ie, severity vs disability and interference) assessment of pain is a particular strength of this study,[35] and an important advancement in the literature. Whereas the self-reported perception of pain severity was essentially unaltered by CBT-I, the extent to which pain reportedly interfered with daily functioning was significantly reduced. One implication of this finding is that CBT-I may be more efficacious for improving the ability to cope with pain rather than perceptions of pain severity/intensity itself.

It seems that, despite minimal changes in the severity of pain, patients are less inclined to perceive pain-related functional limitations following CBT-I. Although the reason for this distinction at present is unclear, the authors speculate that as the perception of pain interference declines, patients may be less likely to experience disability and impairment of social functioning.[39] In turn, this may promote an increase in healthy pain-coping behaviors. Such effects may not translate into pain severity changes in the short term, and the failure of CBT-I to produce short-term changes in pain severity, despite changes in pain interference, is consistent with effects observed in trials of CBT-P, in which pain coping is directly targeted.[26] Thus, longer-term follow-ups in the range of 1 to 2 years may be warranted for these effects to be fully manifested. Such a study would be reasonable given the durability of CBT-I over these longer-term periods, and the general intractability of many chronic pain conditions.

HYBRID CBT-I FOR COMORBID INSOMNIA AND CHRONIC PAIN

If the inconsistency in pain severity changes across CBT-I trials in patients with comorbid insomnia and chronic pain is due to a narrow treatment focus on sleep behaviors and cognitions, it is possible that a hybrid intervention targeting both sleep and pain may produce more favorable results. Given the similarity in theoretical grounding of cognitive and behavioral skills taught in both CBT-I and CBT-P, it is reasonable to hypothesize that a hybrid of the two may be feasibly delivered and more efficiently treat symptoms of both insomnia and pain. Two preliminary pilot studies have examined the effects of a hybrid intervention of CBT-I/CBT-P on pain and insomnia symptoms.

Pigeon and Colleagues

Primary findings
A 10-week hybrid intervention was delivered to patients with chronic noncancer pain and comorbid insomnia.[40] The efficacy of the hybrid intervention (n = 6) was compared with CBT-P alone (n = 5), CBT-I alone (n = 6), and a wait-list control (n = 4) at postintervention, but no follow-up time points. The hybrid intervention contained all components of both the CBT-I and CBT-P conditions (see **Table 1** for complete treatment components). The pain treatment components in both the CBT-P and hybrid conditions included pain psychophysiology education, relaxation training, pacing, pain-specific cognitive therapy, activity planning, problem solving, communication skills, pain flare-up planning, and relapse prevention.[40] The timing

and sequence of specific intervention components was not explicitly described. Results indicated that the largest effect for pain severity was observed in the CBT-P group, whereas the CBT-I and hybrid groups did not show improvements in pain severity (**Table 2**). CBT-P also produced the largest reduction in pain disability, but modest reductions on pain disability were also observed for CBT-I and the hybrid intervention (between-group Cohen d = 0.28 and 0.35, respectively). With respect to insomnia severity, however, the largest effect was observed for the hybrid treatment, followed by CBT-I, and a smaller, nonsignificant effect for CBT-P. The hybrid and CBT-I interventions evidenced similar gains in diary-measured sleep continuity, including approximately 50-minute increases in TST from baseline, and mean SE higher than 90% (from baseline mean <70%) at postintervention, both clinically significant (but not statistically significant) marks.

Analysis

In sum, the findings of this study establish the feasibility of a hybrid insomnia/pain intervention. Across outcomes of both sleep and pain, the hybrid intervention was comparable with CBT-I. Of interest, the hybrid intervention was not efficacious for pain severity and was not significantly different to control for pain disability, despite a modest

reduction. The small sample size, however, precludes any firm conclusions. One interesting aspect of this study is the use of a CBT-P arm, which demonstrated benefits for chronic pain symptoms but failed to alleviate insomnia symptoms. As with the studies reviewed earlier, the findings of Pigeon and colleagues[40] should be cautiously interpreted until a larger study is conducted.

Tang and Colleagues

Primary findings

One other pilot study[41] investigated the effects of a 4-week hybrid intervention (n = 10; see **Table 1** for treatment component details) in comparison with a symptom-monitoring control group (n = 10) in patients with chronic heterogeneous, non-malignant pain and comorbid insomnia. The sleep interventions included stimulus control and sleep-restriction therapies. The pain treatment components in the hybrid intervention included pain education, behavioral activation, and cognitive therapy focused on reducing pain catastrophizing, safety-seeking behavior, and increasing positive reappraisal and growth strategies. Sessions lasted 2 hours, but the sequencing of individual components was not explicitly described. Significant improvements at postintervention were observed for the hybrid intervention relative to the control in

Table 2
Between-group effect size estimates for CBT-I and hybrid interventions on key outcomes after intervention

Authors,[Ref.] Year	Diary SOL	Diary SE	Diary WASO	Diary TST	Pain Severity	Functional Pain Measure
Studies in which CBT-I was the active treatment						
Currie et al,[24] 2000	0.76	1.02	0.94	0.40	0.51	—
Rybarczyk et al,[27] 2005; Vitiello et al,[28] 2009	0.36	0.75	0.89	0.03	0.53	—
Edinger et al,[31] 2005[a]	0.08	0.73	1.51	0.01	0.17	—
Jungquist et al,[35] 2010; Jungquist et al,[38] 2012	2.28	1.95	1.69	1.12	0.81	0.67 (MPI) 1.06 (PDI)
Studies in which hybrid CBT-I/-P was the active treatment						
Pigeon et al,[40] 2012[b]	—	1.48	—	0.66	0.37	0.39 (PDI)
Tang et al,[41] 2012	1.84	1.94	2.10	0.73	0.05	1.34 (BPI)
Vitiello et al,[42] 2013[c]	—	2.64[d]	—		0.10	—

Values are Cohen's d effect-size estimates derived from between-group (treatment vs control) comparisons at posttreatment time points.

Abbreviations: BPI, Brief Pain Inventory, Pain Interference Subscale; MPI, Multidimensional Pain Inventory, Pain Interference Subscale; PDI, Pain Disability Index.

[a] Study included multiple control groups; effect size derived from CBT-I/usual care comparison.
[b] Study included multiple control groups; effect size derived from hybrid/wait-list control comparison.
[c] Study included multiple control groups; effect size derived from hybrid/education control comparison.
[d] Actigraphy was the only modality used to assess SE in this study.

insomnia severity, diary-reported SOL, WASO, SE, and TST (see **Table 2** for between-group effect sizes), in addition to actigraphically assessed SOL, WASO, TST, and TIB. The hybrid intervention was associated with significant postintervention improvements in pain interference but not pain severity. Primary diary and actigraphy measures were not obtained on follow-up, but 1-month and 6-month follow-up data were available for retrospective questionnaire data, which included insomnia severity, pain severity, and interference. Significant pre-post gains in insomnia severity and pain interference were maintained at 1-month and 6-month follow-up.

Vitiello and Colleagues

Primary findings

Vitiello and colleagues[42] reported results from the largest RCT of CBT for comorbid insomnia and chronic pain, with 367 older adults randomized to receive a hybrid CBT-I/P, CBT-P, or an education control. The hybrid intervention resulted in significantly greater reductions in self-reported insomnia severity than either CBT-P or the education control, and these effects were maintained at 9 month follow-up. The only objective sleep outcome reported— actigraphically-measured SE—improved in both CBT-I/P and CBT-P, and declined in the education control group. Neither CBT-I/P nor CBT-P significantly improved in pain severity. Secondary analyses on all primary outcomes in a subgroup of patients with heightened baseline pain did not reveal a substantively different pattern of results.

Analysis

The primary strengths of the Vitiello and colleagues[42] were its large sample size, rigorous design, and excellent retention of participants at 9-month follow-up. The findings support those of Pigeon et al. and Tang et al. in 2 respects. First, all three studies suggest CBT-I/P is efficacious in reducing insomnia severity. Second, all three studies suggest CBT-I/P is not efficacious in reducing pain severity. Together, the data from the studies of Tang and colleagues[41] and Pigeon and colleagues[40] confirm the feasibility of a hybrid intervention. Furthermore, they demonstrate that brief (ie, 4 sessions) and longer (ie, 10 sessions) hybrid intervention formats produce comparable results on sleep outcomes. There was overlap in the content of hybrid interventions in both of these studies (see **Table 1** for comparisons). Relative to the study by Pigeon and colleagues,[40] Tang and colleagues'[41] intervention notably omitted relaxation and relapse prevention modules for both

insomnia and pain. Pigeon and colleagues reported "pain-specific cognitive therapy" as a therapeutic module, but did not provide additional details about the content of the cognitive therapy. By contrast, Tang and colleagues reported incorporating specific modules on positive reappraisal and growth, in addition to cognitive therapy to reduce pain catastrophizing. It is notable that within the intervention of Pigeon and colleagues,[40] the hybrid condition included twice as many components in the same number of sessions as both the CBT-I and CBT-P comparison conditions. Although speculative, it is possible that the absence of hybrid intervention effects on pain severity in this study was due to patient difficulty in managing the demands of simultaneously learning a large number of pain-coping skills and sleep-habit changes. Although Vitiello and colleagues spread their hybrid modules over more sessions, they too failed to find pain reduction following CBT-I/P. It would be interesting to see in future studies whether reducing the number of skills taught improves pain-related outcomes in hybrid interventions (although Pigeon and colleagues[40] noted that patients and therapists anecdotally remarked that the number of sessions could actually be reduced and still accommodate the material). Future hybrid interventions may be better evaluated by measuring process and adherence measures in addition to discrete outcomes. For example, it would be useful to know whether patients adhered to sleep and pain home practice assignments differently in the hybrid intervention when compared with the CBT-I and CBT-P interventions.

INTEGRATED ANALYSIS AND FUTURE DIRECTIONS

The available evidence consistently indicates that cognitive-behavioral interventions targeting sleep in patients with chronic pain, including both stand-alone CBT-I and hybrid CBT-I/CBT-P interventions, are efficacious for a range of outcomes derived from sleep diaries and actigraphy, including sleep duration, continuity, and perceived quality. Furthermore, CBT-I and hybrid interventions may improve pain-related outcomes, with greater effects on pain interference and disability relative to pain severity. The 2 preliminary hybrid interventions incorporating elements of both pain and sleep seem to primarily benefit sleep, with modest effects on pain interference and disability. Despite the promise of these initial findings, they are limited by several factors that must be addressed in future research.

Sample Size

Small sample sizes in the treatment and control conditions of all of the RCTs to date threaten the reliability and validity of the data. Increasing the sample size is the most straightforward way to improve reliability and validity in the outcome data available from existing trials.

Optimization of Sleep Outcome Measurement

A more complex issue than sample size is how to optimize outcome measurement. All RCTs reviewed used daily diaries to assess primary sleep outcomes, and 5 studies[24,31,35,41,42] additionally used actigraphic measurements. In general, the diary procedures are minimally described across studies, and only very limited data pertaining to participant adherence are available across studies. In several studies, it is not clear whether the diaries were paper/pencil or electronic, the latter of which can be objectively verified with time stamps and, therefore, may produce more reliable data. Thus, it is unclear whether diary entries were reliably made within specified windows, and how much retrospective bias may have interfered with self-report estimations. Furthermore, no empirically validated methods are available to guide the analysis of actigraphy data for patients with comorbid insomnia and chronic pain. It is plausible, for example, that patients with certain chronic pain disorders may evidence greater WASO on actigraphy by virtue of heightened motor activity related to the pain source (eg, leg movements due to knee osteoarthritis). This pattern was observed in the study by Jungquist and colleagues,[38] in which actigraphy-assessed WASO was significantly greater than daily diary–assessed WASO. By contrast, Edinger and colleagues[31] did not report any systematic differences between diary-based and actigraphy-based outcomes. Future research should examine the validity of actigraphy as an outcome measure by determining whether actigraphically assessed sleep parameters are different in patients with certain types of chronic pain. As ambulatory polysomnography (PSG) becomes increasingly available and affordable, the reliability and validity of actigraphy data may be readily compared with those of PSG.

Optimization of Pain Outcome Measurement

Though interpreted with caution because of small sample sizes, the available data suggest that pain severity may not be robustly altered by CBT-I and hybrid CBT-I/CBT-P, and therefore may be a poor primary end point, at least when measured within 6 months. Other more functionally relevant outcomes, such as pain interference, seem to be more strongly influenced by CBT-I and hybrid interventions.[35,41] The minimal effects on pain severity contrast with those in the experimental literature because they suggest that changes in sleep do not precipitate changes in pain. However, an alternative explanation is that the pain assessments in clinical trials to date have not been sufficiently broad to capture the true variance or complexities underpinning the association of insomnia with chronic pain. For example, in future studies it may prove important to incorporate a broader range of diary-based pain-related outcomes and to evaluate time-variant contingencies in pain, sleep, functional disability, mood, and stress from day to day.[43,44] Such an assessment strategy would yield potentially important information about the psychosocial antecedents and sequelae of changes in pain and sleep from one day to the next, and whether such contingent daily associations change following treatment. In addition, it may be useful to investigate individual differences in response to quantitative sensory testing (QST). QST includes a range of nociceptive stimuli (eg, thermal, pressure, electrodermal) that evoke a variable range of pain responses in individuals with and without chronic pain.[8] Experimental studies have demonstrated that response to QST, including pain threshold[45–48] and endogenous pain inhibition,[49] are altered by sleep deprivation. The evaluation of changes in QST responses throughout treatment may shed light on the ability of CBT-I to effect change on neurobiologically mediated processes that may contribute to the maintenance of chronic pain, such as central sensitization[50,51] and endogenous pain inhibition.[52] The mechanisms by which such changes may take place are not clear at present, although sleep has been identified as a potential source of variance in these endogenous pain modulatory processes.[49,53] In addition, physical function and psychosocial factors are associated with dysfunctional endogenous pain modulation.[50,54] If CBT-I and hybrid interventions are shown to reliably improve sleep and functional pain-related outcomes, it is reasonable to postulate that such effects may be associated with improved endogenous pain modulation, which might be hypothesized to precede changes in clinical pain reporting. The potential for such changes to affect clinical pain severity might be best determined over long-term follow-up (eg, 1–3 years), and therefore may not be reflected in the results of the studies reviewed here.

Examination of Demographic Moderators

Many of the studies reviewed were not large enough to investigate or explore the possibility that key moderators known to influence pain sensitivity and sleep, such as sex, age, and ethnicity,[55–60] may have obscured the effects. Although the Vitiello and colleagues study was powered to explore such effects, they did not report them in their initial publication. Future studies should examine these moderation models. It is possible, for example, that demographic subgroups vary in the magnitude or time course of response to CBT-I and/or a hybrid intervention.

Evaluation of Secondary Sleep-Related Phenomena

Another potentially important issue that creates complexity within this literature is the possibility that other sleep-related phenomena, such as central or obstructive apneas and periodic limb movements (PLMs), may influence some of the pain-related outcomes. Although all studies reviewed here attempted to identify many of these intrinsic sleep disorders for the purpose of exclusion through self-report (eg, Structured Interview for Sleep Disorders), 3 studies[24,41,42] did not use polysomnography to rule out sleep disorders other than insomnia, and the remaining studies varied in the thresholds used to exclude subjects based on apnea-hypopnea index (AHI; number of apneas and hypopneas per hour of sleep) and PLM index (number of PLMs per hour of sleep) (see **Table 1**). It is likely that severe cases of sleep apnea and PLM disorder were excluded from the studies, but it is possible that variability among individuals with mild apnea (eg, AHI 5–15) and PLMs (eg, PLM index <15) may have influenced results. None of the studies reviewed attempted to control or assess the effect of these indices on outcomes. However, emerging data suggest, for example, that sleep-related hypoxemia may actually reduce pain sensitivity in patients with chronic pain.[61,62] Other data suggest that nocturnal hypoxemia may increase pain sensitivity, especially in healthy subjects.[63] Thus, future studies should covary continuous measures of hypoxemia and other relevant nocturnal phenomena to partial out any potential influence on primary outcomes.

Process-Oriented Evaluation of Hybrid Intervention Components

Theoretically, hybrid interventions may offer advantages over CBT-I for pain outcomes by incorporating strategies to behaviorally manage both sleep and pain.[64] Future hybrid studies may yet bear this out, as the effect sizes of CBT-I on pain severity are comparable with the effects of CBT-P on pain severity. However, at present it seems that findings in the experimental[7,14,45,48,49,65] and longitudinal literature[13,53,66,67] that support a causal association between sleep and pain severity may not easily translate into the treatment context in this first wave of studies. That said, it may simply be the case that a more systematic refinement of hybrid treatment protocols may be needed to yield treatment gains. Issues related to the sequencing of pain-related and sleep-related treatment components may be critical and have yet to be investigated. It may additionally be necessary to evaluate which sleep and pain components are the most compatible, and whether specific pairings of sleep and pain components enhances or detracts from outcomes. It is possible that flooding patients with too many skills over too short a period of time may have contributed to the relatively disappointing preliminary findings, particularly with respect to the study by Pigeon and colleagues.[40] Tang and colleagues'[41] intervention incorporated fewer treatment components, but needs to be tested against CBT-I and CBT-P with long-term follow-up to understand its true promise.

Larger-scale investigations of CBT-I in patients with comorbid insomnia and chronic pain are currently under way. An ongoing RCT in the authors' laboratory is comparing the effects of CBT-I with those of an active placebo (behavioral desensitization) on clinical pain and QST in patients with knee osteoarthritis and comorbid insomnia.

SUMMARY

Insomnia and chronic pain harbor a high rate of comorbidity, and have been regarded as reciprocally related conditions. Four RCTs have investigated the efficacy of CBT-I and 2 RCTs have investigated the efficacy of hybrid CBT-I/CBT-P interventions in reducing insomnia and pain symptoms. In general, these interventions demonstrate clinically meaningful improvements in sleep symptoms. Improvements in pain-related outcomes have been observed in functional domains, such as pain interference and disability, with limited evidence supporting the short-term efficacy of CBT-I or hybrid interventions for pain severity. Hybrid interventions are feasible, and one large-scale RCT now supports the findings of 2 pilot studies, suggesting that hybrid interventions, as currently designed, improve sleep, but not pain severity. Future clinical trials should consider using more comprehensive pain assessments with longer-term follow-up assessment of at least 1 year or more. Measurement strategies that permit the analysis of time-variant contingencies in sleep, pain, and associated psychosocial variables may also be particularly informative. Larger-scale investigations are needed to clarify the limited efficacy data from the small pilot RCTs on hybrid interventions. Future studies aimed at developing hybrid interventions should be designed to investigate issues related to the sequencing of pain and sleep components, and should address the trade-off between the number of new skills patients are expected to master and the quality and mastery of critical components. Hybrid approaches that combine sleep and pain intervention components continue to hold promise for improving the treatment of chronic pain among patients with comorbid insomnia.

REFERENCES

1. Irwin M, McClintick J, Costlow C, et al. Partial night sleep deprivation reduces natural killer and cellular immune responses in humans. FASEB J 1996; 10(5):643–53.

2. Mullington JM, Haack M, Toth M, et al. Cardiovascular, inflammatory and metabolic consequences of sleep deprivation. Prog Cardiovasc Dis 2009; 51(4):294.

3. Yoo SS, Gujar N, Hu P, et al. The human emotional brain without sleep: a prefrontal amygdala disconnect. Curr Biol 2007;17(20):R877–8.

4. Zohar D, Tzischinsky O, Epstein R, et al. The effects of sleep loss on medical residents' emotional reactions to work events: a cognitive-energy model. Sleep 2005;28(1):47–54.

5. Durmer JS, Dinges DF. Neurocognitive consequences of sleep deprivation. Semin Neurol 2005; 25(1):117–29.

6. Thomas M, Sing H, Belenky G, et al. Neural basis of alertness and cognitive performance impairments during sleepiness. I. Effects of 24 h of sleep deprivation on waking human regional brain activity. J Sleep Res 2000;9(4):335–52.

7. Lautenbacher S, Kundermann B, Krieg JC. Sleep deprivation and pain perception. Sleep Med Rev 2006;10(5):357–69.

8. Edwards RR, Sarlani E, Wesselmann U, et al. Quantitative assessment of experimental pain perception: multiple domains of clinical relevance. Pain 2005;114(3):315–9.

9. Lumley MA, Cohen JL, Borszcz GS, et al. Pain and emotion: a biopsychosocial review of recent research. J Clin Psychol 2011;67(9):942–68.

10. Marchand F, Perretti M, McMahon SB. Role of the immune system in chronic pain. Nat Rev Neurosci 2005;6(7):521–32.

11. Weiner DK, Rudy TE, Morrow L, et al. The relationship between pain, neuropsychological performance, and physical function in community-dwelling older adults with chronic low back pain. Pain Med 2006;7(1): 60–70.

12. Williams AC, Eccleston C, Morley S. Psychological therapies for the management of chronic pain (excluding headache) in adults. Cochrane Database Syst Rev 2012;(11):CD007407.

13. Quartana PJ, Wickwire EM, Klick B, et al. Naturalistic changes in insomnia symptoms and pain in temporomandibular joint disorder: a cross-lagged panel analysis. Pain 2010;149(2):325–31.

14. Roehrs TA, Harris E, Randall S, et al. Pain sensitivity and recovery from mild chronic sleep loss. Sleep 2012;35(12):1667–72.

15. Morin CM, Colecchi C, Stone J, et al. Behavioral and pharmacological therapies for late-life insomnia. JAMA 1999;281(11):991–9.

16. Morin CM, Valleres A, Guay B, et al. Cognitive behavioral therapy, singly and combined with medication, for persistent insomnia. JAMA 2009; 301(19):2005–15.

17. Sivertsen B, Krokstad S, Overland S, et al. The epidemiology of insomnia: associations with physical and mental health. The HUNT-2 study. J Psychosom Res 2009;67(2):109–16.

18. Bastien CH, Morin CM, Ouellet MC, et al. Cognitive-behavioral therapy for insomnia: comparison of individual therapy, group therapy, and telephone consultations. J Consult Clin Psychol 2004;72(4):653.

19. Edinger JD, Sampson WS. A primary care "friendly" cognitive behavioral insomnia therapy. Sleep 2003;26(2):177–84.

20. Backhaus J, Hohagen F, Voderholzer U, et al. Long-term effectiveness of a short-term cognitive-behavioral group treatment for primary insomnia. Eur Arch Psychiatry Clin Neurosci 2001;251(1):35–41.

21. Manber R, Edinger JD, Gress JL, et al. Cognitive behavioral therapy for insomnia enhances depression outcome in patients with comorbid major depressive disorder and insomnia. Sleep 2008; 31(4):489.

22. Smith MT, Huang MI, Manber R. Cognitive behavior therapy for chronic insomnia occurring within the context of medical and psychiatric disorders. Clin Psychol Rev 2005;25(5):559–92.

23. Spielman AJ, Saskin P, Thorpy MJ. Treatment of chronic insomnia by restriction of time in bed. Sleep 1987;10(1):45–56.

24. Currie SR, Wilson KG, Pontefract AJ, et al. Cognitive-behavioral treatment of insomnia secondary to chronic pain. J Consult Clin Psychol 2000; 68(3):407.

25. Cohen J. Statistical power analysis for the behavioral sciences. 2nd edition. Hillsdale (NJ): Erlbaum; 1988.

26. Morley S, Eccleston C, Williams A. Systematic review and meta-analysis of randomized controlled trials of cognitive behaviour therapy and behaviour therapy for chronic pain in adults, excluding headache. Pain 1999;80(1):1–13.

27. Rybarczyk B, Stepanski E, Fogg L, et al. A placebo-controlled test of cognitive-behavioral therapy for comorbid insomnia in older adults. J Consult Clin Psychol 2005;73(6):1164.

28. Vitiello MV, Rybarczyk B, Von Korff M, et al. Cognitive behavioral therapy for insomnia improves sleep and decreases pain in older adults with comorbid insomnia and osteoarthritis. J Clin Sleep Med 2009;5(4):355.

29. Melzack R. The short-form McGill pain questionnaire. Pain 1987;30(2):191–7.

30. Ware JE, Kosinski M, Keller S. SF-36 physical and mental health summary scales: a user's manual. Health Assessment Lab; 1994.

31. Edinger JD, Wohlgemuth WK, Krystal AD, et al. Behavioral insomnia therapy for fibromyalgia patients: a randomized clinical trial. Arch Intern Med 2005;165(21):2527.

32. Cleeland CS, Ryan KM. Pain assessment: global use of the Brief Pain Inventory. Ann Acad Med Singapore 1994;23(2):129.

33. Burckhardt CS, Clark SR, Bennett RM. The fibromyalgia impact questionnaire: development and validation. J Rheumatol 1991;18(5):728–33.

34. Roizenblatt S, Neto NS, Tufik S. Sleep disorders and fibromyalgia. Curr Pain Headache Rep 2011; 15(5):347–57.

35. Jungquist CR, O'Brien C, Matteson-Rusby S, et al. The efficacy of cognitive-behavioral therapy for insomnia in patients with chronic pain. Sleep Med 2010;11(3):302–9.

36. Kerns RD, Turk DC, Rudy TE. The West Haven-Yale Multidimensional Pain Inventory (WHYMPI). Pain 1985;23(4):345–56.

37. Chibnall JT, Tait RC. The Pain Disability Index: factor structure and normative data. Arch Phys Med Rehabil 1994;75(10):1082.

38. Jungquist CR, Tra Y, Smith MT, et al. The durability of cognitive behavioral therapy for insomnia in patients with chronic pain. Sleep Disord 2012;2012: 679648.

39. Wittink H, Turk DC, Carr DB, et al. Comparison of the redundancy, reliability, and responsiveness to change among SF-36, Oswestry Disability Index, and Multidimensional Pain Inventory. Clin J Pain 2004;20(3):133–42.

40. Pigeon WR, Moynihan J, Matteson-Rusby S, et al. Comparative effectiveness of CBT interventions for co-morbid chronic pain & insomnia: a pilot study. Behav Res Ther 2012;50:685–9.

41. Tang NK, Goodchild CE, Salkovskis PM. Hybrid cognitive-behaviour therapy for individuals with insomnia and chronic pain: a pilot randomised controlled trial. Behav Res Ther 2012;50:814–21.

42. Vitiello MV, McCurry SM, Shortreed SM, et al. Cognitive-behavioral treatment for comorbid insomnia and osteoarthritis pian in primary care: The Lifestyles Randomized Controlled Trial. Journal of the American Geriatrics Society 2013;61:947–56.

43. Davis MC, Zautra AJ, Smith BW. Chronic pain, stress, and the dynamics of affective differentiation. J Pers 2004;72(6):1133–59.

44. Zautra AJ, Affleck GG, Tennen H, et al. Dynamic approaches to emotions and stress in everyday life: Bolger and Zuckerman reloaded with positive as well as negative affects. J Pers 2005;73(6):1511–38.

45. Kundermann B, Spernal J, Huber MT, et al. Sleep deprivation affects thermal pain thresholds but not somatosensory thresholds in healthy volunteers. Psychosom Med 2004;66(6):932–7.

46. Lentz MJ, Landis CA, Rothermel J, et al. Effects of selective slow wave sleep disruption on musculoskeletal pain and fatigue in middle aged women. J Rheumatol 1999;26(7):1586.

47. Onen SH, Alloui A, Gross A, et al. The effects of total sleep deprivation, selective sleep interruption and sleep recovery on pain tolerance thresholds in healthy subjects. J Sleep Res 2001;10(1):35–42.

48. Roehrs T, Hyde M, Blaisdell B, et al. Sleep loss and REM sleep loss are hyperalgesic. Sleep 2006; 29(2):145.

49. Smith MT, Edwards RR, McCann UD, et al. The effects of sleep deprivation on pain inhibition and spontaneous pain in women. Sleep 2007;30(4): 494–505.

50. Edwards RR, Smith MT, Stonerock G, et al. Pain-related catastrophizing in healthy women is associated with greater temporal summation of and reduced habituation to thermal pain. Clin J Pain 2006;22(8):730–7.

51. Girbes EL, Nijs J, Torres-Cueco R, et al. Pain treatment for patients with osteoarthritis and central sensitization. Phys Ther 2013;93:842–51.

52. Yarnitsky D. Conditioned pain modulation (the diffuse noxious inhibitory control-like effect): its relevance for acute and chronic pain states. Curr Opin Anaesthesiol 2010;23(5):611–5.

53. Edwards RR, Grace E, Peterson S, et al. Sleep continuity and architecture: associations with pain-inhibitory processes in patients with temporomandibular joint disorder. Eur J Pain 2009;13(10): 1043–7.

54. Edwards RR, Ness TJ, Weigent DA, et al. Individual differences in diffuse noxious inhibitory controls (DNIC): association with clinical variables. Pain 2003;106(3):427–37.

55. Durrence HH, Lichstein KL. The sleep of African Americans: a comparative review. Behav Sleep Med 2006;4(1):29–44.

56. Foley D, Ancoli-Israel S, Britz P, et al. Sleep disturbances and chronic disease in older adults: results
of the 2003 National Sleep Foundation Sleep in America Survey. J Psychosom Res 2004;56(5):497–502.

57. Mogil JS. Sex differences in pain and pain inhibition: multiple explanations of a controversial phenomenon. Nat Rev Neurosci 2012;13(12):859–66.

58. Ohayon MM, Carskadon MA, Guilleminault C, et al.
Meta-analysis of quantitative sleep parameters
from childhood to old age in healthy individuals:
developing normative sleep values across the
human lifespan. Sleep 2004;27(7):1255–73.

59. Song Y, Ancoli-Israel S, Lewis CE, et al. The association of race/ethnicity with objectively measured
sleep characteristics in older men. Behav Sleep
Med 2011;10(1):54–69.

60. Zhang B, Wing Y. Sex differences in insomnia: a
meta-analysis. Sleep 2006;29(1):85.

61. Lovati C, Zardoni M, D'Amico D, et al. Possible relationships between headache—allodynia and
nocturnal sleep breathing. Neurol Sci 2011;32(1):
145–8.

62. Smith MT, Wickwire EM, Grace EG, et al. Sleep disorders and their association with laboratory pain
sensitivity in temporomandibular joint disorder.
Sleep 2009;32(6):779.

63. Onen S, Onen F, Albrand G, et al. Pain tolerance
and obstructive sleep apnea in the elderly. J Am
Med Dir Assoc 2010;11(9):612–6.

64. Tang NK. Cognitive-behavioral therapy for sleep
abnormalities of chronic pain patients. Curr Rheumatol Rep 2009;11(6):451–60.

65. Irwin MR, Olmstead R, Carrillo C, et al. Sleep loss
exacerbates fatigue, depression, and pain in rheu-
matoid arthritis. Sleep 2012;35(4):537.

66. Lewandowski AS, Palermo TM, De la Motte S, et al.
Temporal daily associations between pain and
sleep in adolescents with chronic pain versus
healthy adolescents. Pain 2010;151(1):220.

67. Tang NK, Goodchild CE, Sanborn AN, et al. Deci-
phering the temporal link between pain and sleep
in a heterogeneous chronic pain patient sample:
a multilevel daily process study. Sleep 2012;
35(5):675.

Index

Note: Page numbers of article titles are in **boldface** type.

Sleep Med Clin 9 (2014) 275–279
http://dx.doi.org/10.1016/S1556-407X(14)00039-3
1556-407X/14/$ – see front matter © 2014 Elsevier Inc. All rights reserved.

sleep.theclinics.com

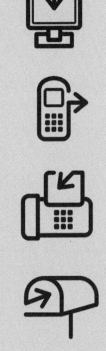

Printed and bound by CPI Group (UK) Ltd, Croydon, CR0 4YY

03/10/2024

01040379-0010